NCLEX-RN

250 New-Format Questions

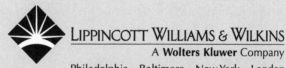

LIPPINCOTT WILLIAMS & WILKINS
A **Wolters Kluwer** Company

Philadelphia • Baltimore • New York • London
Buenos Aires • Hong Kong • Sydney • Tokyo

STAFF

Publisher
Judith A. Schilling McCann, RN, MSN

Editorial Director
David Moreau

Clinical Director
Joan M. Robinson, RN, MSN

Senior Art Director
Arlene Putterman

Editors
Jaime L. Stockslager (senior editor), Tracy S. Diehl (senior associate editor), Kevin Haworth, Barbara Hodgson, Brenna H. Mayer, Liz Schaeffer, Pam Wingrod

Clinical Editors
Lisa Morris Bonsall, RN, MSN, CRNP; Marcy Caplin, RN, MSN; Collette Hendler, RN, BS, CCRN; Anita Lockhart, RNC, MSN; Barbara Stiebeling, RN, MSN

Copy Editor
Kimberly Bilotta

Designer
Lynn Foulk (project manager)

Digital Composition Services
Diane Paluba (manager), Joyce Rossi Biletz (senior desktop assistant), Donna S. Morris (senior desktop assistant)

Manufacturing
Patricia K. Dorshaw (senior manager), Beth Janae Orr (book production coordinator)

Editorial Assistants
Megan Lane Aldinger, Tara Carter-Bell, Arlene P. Claffee, Linda Ruhf

RN250 — D N O S A J J
05 04   10 9 8 7 6 5 4 3

Library of Congress Cataloging-in-Publication Data

NCLEX-RN 250 new-format questions : preparing for the revised NCLEX-RN.
   p. ; cm.
   1. Nursing — Examinations, questions, etc. 2. Nursing — Outlines, syllabi, etc. 3. Nurses — Licenses — United States — Examinations — Study guides. [DNLM: 1. Nursing Care — Examination Questions. 2. Nursing — Examination Questions. WY 18.2 N339 2004] I. Lippincott Williams & Wilkins.

RT55.N435 2004
610.73'076 — dc21
ISBN 1-58255-307-6 (pbk.: alk. paper)   2003013188

Contents

Contributors

Adrianne E. Avillion, RN, D.Ed
President
AEA Consulting
York, Pa.

Peggy D. Baikie, RN,C, MS, NNP, PNP
Senior Instructor-Nurse Practitioner
School of Nursing
University of Colorado Health Sciences Center
Denver

Lisa Morris Bonsall, RN, MSN, CRNP
Independent Clinical Consultant
West Chester, Pa.

Barbara Broome, RN, PhD, CNS
Assistant Dean
Chair of Community Mental Health
College of Nursing
University of South Alabama
Mobile, Ala.

Colleen C. Burgess, RN, MSN, APRN, BC, NCSAC
Department Head of Nursing
Catawba Valley Community College
Hickory, N.C.

Michelle M. Byrne, RN, PhD, CNOR
Clinical Faculty
North Georgia College & State University
Dahlonega, Ga.

Joseph T. Catalano, RN, PhD
Professor and Chairman
Department of Nursing
East Central University
Ada, Okla.

Kathleen Clark, RN, MSN, APR, BC, CNRN
Nursing Faculty
Thomas Jefferson University
Philadelphia

Marsha L. Conroy, RN, MSN, APN
Nurse Educator
Cuyahoga Community College
Cleveland
Kent (Ohio) State University

Linda Carman Copel, RN, PhD, CS, DAPA
Associate Professor
College of Nursing
Villanova (Pa.) University

Shelba Durston, RN, MSN, CCRN
Adjunct Faculty
San Joaquin Delta College
Stockton, Calif.
Staff Nurse—Intensive Care Unit
San Joaquin General Hospital
French Camp, Calif.

Athena Foreman, RN, MSN
Senior Level Nursing Coordinator
Stanly Community College
Albemarle, N.C.

Elaine L. Gross, RN, MSN
Assistant Professor
Temple University
Philadelphia

Nancy H. Haynes, RN, MN, CCRN
Assistant Professor of Nursing
Saint Luke's College
Kansas City, Mo.

Jacqueline M. Lamb, RN, PhD
Assistant Professor
School of Nursing
University of Pittsburgh

Nan Riede, RN, MSN
Assistant Professor
Baptist College of Health Sciences
Memphis

Matthew R. Sorenson, RN, PhD
Post-Doctoral Nursing Fellow
Edward Hines Jr. VA Hospital
Hines, Ill.

Preface

You've worked hard to earn your degree. You're ready to move ahead in your career and begin your nursing practice. Only one thing stands in your way — the National Council Licensure Examination for Registered Nurses (NCLEX-RN). Every nursing student is familiar with the pressure and anxiety involved with taking the NCLEX-RN. As if the stress of the standard test questions weren't enough, however, the National Council of State Boards of Nursing (NCSBN) recently added three types of alternate item questions to the NCLEX. But don't worry, *NCLEX-RN: 250 New-Format Questions* is a cutting-edge review book that will help you become fully prepared for every type of question you may encounter on the NCLEX.

The first type of alternate item format is the multiple-response multiple-choice question. Unlike a traditional multiple-choice question, each multiple-response multiple-choice question has more than one correct answer, and it may contain more than four possible answer options. You'll recognize this type of question because you'll be asked to select **all** answers that apply — not just the **best** answer (as may be requested in the more traditional multiple-choice questions).

When you encounter one of these questions in this review book, read the question and all possible answers carefully. Place a check mark in the box next to all options that correctly answer the question. Keep in mind that, for each multiple-response multiple-choice question, you must select **at least two answers** and you must select **all correct answers** for the item to be counted as correct. On the NCLEX, there is no partial credit in the scoring of these items.

The second type of alternate item format is the fill-in-the-blank. These questions require you to provide the answer yourself, rather than select it from a list of options. For these questions, write your answer in the blank space provided after the question. Keep in mind that the computerized version of the NCLEX may require that you type in a very specific response in order for it to be considered correct (for example, "Mammography" rather than "Mammogram").

For purposes of this review, be as specific as possible with each of your answers to fill-in-the-blank questions. The answers we've supplied are the short-est, most precise responses, although, as noted above, variations may be possible. The NCSBN has not yet made clear how it will handle such variations on possible answers on its computerized test.

The third and final type of alternate item format is a question in which you will be asked to identify an area on an illustration or graphic. For these so-called "Hot spot" questions, the computerized exam will ask you to place your cursor over the correct area on an illustration.

When reviewing such questions in this book, read the question and then mark an X on the illustration in the left-hand column to indicate your answer. In the right-hand column, correct answers are similarly indicated by an X on the duplicate illustration. Try to be as precise as possible when marking the location. As with the fill-in-the-blanks, the identification questions on the computerized exam may require extremely precise answers in order for them to be considered correct.

These new alternate item formats are sure to make the NCLEX exam even more challenging than it has been in the past. Luckily, *NCLEX-RN: 250 New-Format Questions* was specifically developed to help you prepare for and excel at each of these types of questions. This helpful review book will boost your confidence and ease your anxiety.

A useful supplementary study guide, this book includes 250 alternate-format questions that cover all of the topics tested on the exam—including fundamentals of nursing, medical-surgical nursing, maternal-infant nursing, pediatric nursing, and psychiatric and mental health nursing. For each type of question, you'll find the correct answer as well as clear, concise rationales for correct and incorrect answers. You'll also find the associated nursing process step, client needs category and subcategory, and cognitive level.

The convenient two-column format (with questions on the left and answers on the right) enhances your preparation process by giving you instant feedback and saves you the time of flipping to the back of the book to find the correct answer.

The review questions provided in this book will test your knowledge base and improve your test-taking skills as well as help you become familiar with the format of the new questions. All of the questions were written by nurses and approximate the real questions you'll find on the NCLEX.

The NCSBN has not yet established a percentage of alternate item formats to be administered to each candidate. In fact, your exam may contain only one alternate item format. Be confident in knowing that the questions in this book cover relevant information in a challenging format that can be useful even if your NCLEX examination does not include these new format questions. Also, in your rush to prepare for the new format questions, don't forget to review practice questions that follow the standard four-option, multiple-choice format. These questions will still compose the bulk of the test.

Remember that the process of testing and introducing new alternate-format questions into the NCLEX is ongoing. Because the test format is subject to change, be sure to consult the "Testing services" section of the NCSBN web site (*www.ncsbn.org*) as your exam date nears for the most up-to-date information on the NCLEX.

You've been diligently preparing for this all-important exam for years. *NCLEX-RN: 250 New-Format Questions* is the next logical extension of that sound preparation, the final resource you need to meet the challenge of passing NCLEX and moving on to the rewards of your nursing career. Good luck.

Part 1
Fundamentals of nursing

1. The nurse is developing a care plan for a client with injury to the frontal lobe of the brain. Which of the following interventions should be part of the care plan?

Select all that apply:

☐ **A.** Keep instructions simple and brief because the client will have difficulty concentrating.

☐ **B.** Speak clearly and slowly because the client will have difficulty hearing.

☐ **C.** Assist the client with bathing because he will have vision disturbances.

☐ **D.** Orient the client to person, place, and time as needed because of memory problems.

☐ **E.** Assess vital signs frequently since vital bodily functions are affected.

ANSWER: A, D

Rationale: Damage to the frontal lobe affects personality, memory, reasoning, concentration, and motor control of speech. Damage to the temporal lobe, not the frontal lobe, causes hearing and speech problems. Damage to the occipital lobe causes vision disturbances. Damage to the brain stem affects vital functions.

Nursing process step: Planning

Client needs category: Physiological integrity

Client needs subcategory: Basic care and comfort

Cognitive level: Application

2. The nurse is caring for a client with emphysema. Which of the following nursing interventions are appropriate?

Select all that apply:

☐ **A.** Reduce fluid intake to less than 2,500 ml/day.

☐ **B.** Teach diaphragmatic, pursed-lip breathing.

☐ **C.** Administer low-flow oxygen.

☐ **D.** Keep the client in a supine position as much as possible.

☐ **E.** Encourage alternating activity with rest periods.

☐ **F.** Teach use of postural drainage and chest physiotherapy.

ANSWER: B, C, E, F

Rationale: Diaphragmatic, pursed-lip breathing strengthens respiratory muscles and enhances oxygenation in clients with emphysema. Low-flow oxygen should be administered because a client with emphysema has chronic hypercapnia and a hypoxic respiratory drive. Alternating activity with rest allows the client to perform activities without excessive distress. If the client has copious secretions and has difficulty mobilizing secretions, the nurse should teach him and his family members how to perform postural drainage and chest physiotherapy. Fluid intake should be increased to 3,000 ml/day, if not contraindicated, to liquefy secretions and facilitate their removal. The client should be placed in high-Fowler's position to improve ventilation.

Nursing process step: Planning

Client needs category: Physiological integrity

Client needs subcategory: Basic care and comfort

Cognitive level: Application

3. The nurse is caring for a client who underwent surgical repair of a detached retina of the right eye. Which of the following interventions should the nurse perform?

Select all that apply:

☐ **A.** Place the client in a prone position.

☐ **B.** Approach the client from the left side.

☐ **C.** Encourage deep breathing and coughing.

☐ **D.** Discourage bending down.

☐ **E.** Orient the client to his environment.

☐ **F.** Administer a stool softener.

ANSWER: B, D, E, F

Rationale: The nurse should approach the client from the left side — the unaffected side — to avoid startling him. She should also discourage the client from bending down, deep breathing, hard coughing and sneezing, and other activities that can increase intraocular pressure. The client should be oriented to his environment to reduce the risk of injury. Stool softeners should be administered to discourage straining during defecation. The client should lie on his back or on the unaffected side to reduce intraocular pressure on the affected eye.

Nursing process step: Implementation

Client needs category: Physiological integrity

Client needs subcategory: Reduction of risk potential

Cognitive level: Application

---

4. The nurse is planning care for a client with hyperthyroidism. Which of the following nursing interventions are appropriate?

Select all that apply:

☐ **A.** Instill isotonic eye drops, as necessary.

☐ **B.** Provide several small, well-balanced meals.

☐ **C.** Provide rest periods.

☐ **D.** Keep the environment warm.

☐ **E.** Encourage frequent visitors and conversation.

☐ **F.** Weigh the client daily.

ANSWER: A, B, C, F

Rationale: If the client has exophthalmos (a sign of hyperthyroidism), the conjunctivae should be moistened often with isotonic eye drops. Hyperthyroidism results in increased appetite, which can be satisfied by frequent small, well-balanced meals. The nurse should provide the client with rest periods to reduce metabolic demands. The client should be weighed daily to check for weight loss, a possible consequence of hyperthyroidism. Because metabolism is increased in hyperthyroidism, heat intolerance and excitability result. Therefore, the nurse should provide a cool and quiet environment, not a warm and busy one, to promote client comfort.

Nursing process step: Planning

Client needs category: Physiological integrity

Client needs subcategory: Basic care and comfort

Cognitive level: Application

5. The nurse is caring for a client with a hiatal hernia. The client complains of abdominal pain and sternal pain after eating. The pain makes it difficult for him to sleep. Which of the following instructions should the nurse recommend when teaching this client?

Select all that apply:

☐ **A.** Avoid constrictive clothing.

☐ **B.** Lie down for 30 minutes after eating.

☐ **C.** Decrease intake of caffeine and spicy foods.

☐ **D.** Eat three meals per day.

☐ **E.** Sleep in semi-Fowler's position.

☐ **F.** Maintain a normal body weight.

ANSWER: A, C, E, F

Rationale: To reduce gastric reflux, the nurse should instruct the client to sleep with his upper body elevated; lose weight, if obese; avoid constrictive clothing, caffeine, and spicy foods; remain upright for 2 hours after eating; and eat small, frequent meals.

Nursing process step: Implementation

Client needs category: Physiological integrity

Client needs subcategory: Basic care and comfort

Cognitive level: Application

---

6. The client has a tumor of the posterior pituitary gland. The nurse planning his care should include which of the following interventions?

Select all that apply:

☐ **A.** Take daily weight.

☐ **B.** Restrict fluids.

☐ **C.** Assess urine specific gravity.

☐ **D.** Encourage intake of coffee or tea.

☐ **E.** Monitor intake and output.

ANSWER: A, C, E

Rationale: Tumors of the pituitary gland can lead to diabetes insipidus due to deficiency of antidiuretic hormone (ADH). Decreased ADH reduces the ability of the kidneys to concentrate urine, resulting in excessive urination, excessive thirst, and excessive fluid intake. To monitor fluid balance, weigh the client daily, measure urine specific gravity, and monitor intake and output. Encourage fluids to keep intake equal to output and prevent dehydration. Coffee, tea, and other fluids that have a diuretic effect should be avoided.

Nursing process step: Planning

Client needs category: Physiological integrity

Client needs subcategory: Basic care and comfort

Cognitive level: Application

7. A client is blind in the right eye. From which side should the nurse approach the client?

_____

Answer: Left

Rationale: The nurse should approach the client from the left side so that the client can be aware of the nurse's approach. Likewise, personal items should be placed on the client's left side so that he can see them easily.

Nursing process step: Planning

Client needs category: Physiological care

Client needs subcategory: Basic care and comfort

Cognitive level: Comprehension

---

8. The nurse is preparing to boost a client up in bed and instructs the client to use the overbed trapeze. Which risk factor for pressure ulcer development is the nurse reducing by instructing the client to move in this manner?

_____

Answer: Shearing forces

Rationale: Shearing forces (opposing forces that cause layers of skin to move over each other, stretching and tearing capillaries and, eventually, resulting in necrosis) increase the risk of pressure ulcer development. They can occur as clients slide down in bed or are pulled up in bed. Subcutaneous skin layers adhere to the sheets while deeper layers, muscle, and bone slide in the direction of movement. To reduce shearing forces, the nurse should instruct the client to use an overbed trapeze, place a draw sheet under the client to move the client up in bed, and keep the head of the bed no higher than 30 degrees.

Nursing process step: Implementation

Client needs category: Physiological integrity

Client needs subcategory: Basic care and comfort

Cognitive level: Application

9. The nurse is assisting a client with lower motor neuron damage who has difficulty with urination. The nurse shows the client how to apply gentle pressure over the lower abdomen to empty the bladder. By what name does the nurse refer to this procedure?

_____

ANSWER: Credé's maneuver

Rationale: Credé's maneuver is performed by applying manual pressure over the lower abdomen. This procedure promotes complete emptying of the bladder in clients with lower motor neuron damage that impairs the voiding reflex.

Nursing process step: Implementation

Client needs category: Physiological integrity

Client needs subcategory: Basic care and comfort

Cognitive level: Application

10. A postoperative client receives a lunch tray with milk, custard, and vanilla ice cream. What is the client's current diet order?

_____

ANSWER: Full liquid diet

Rationale: A full liquid diet consists of fluids and foods that are liquid at room temperature. Some examples are milk, custard, ice cream, puddings, vegetable and fruit juices, refined or strained cereals, and egg substitutes. A full liquid diet also includes all foods allowed on a clear liquid diet.

Nursing process step: Implementation

Client needs category: Physiological integrity

Client needs subcategory: Basic care and comfort

Cognitive level: Comprehension

11. The nurse is teaching a client with left leg weakness to walk with a cane. The nurse instructs the client to hold the cane in which hand?

_____

Rationale: To ambulate safely, a client with a leg weakness should hold the cane in the hand opposite the weak leg. Because this client has left leg weakness, the cane should be held in the right hand.

Nursing process step: Implementation

Client needs category: Physiological integrity

Client needs subcategory: Basic care and comfort

Cognitive level: Comprehension

12. A client is performing quadriceps sets to strengthen the muscles used for walking. When performing these exercises, the client contracts his quadriceps with no change in muscle length and no joint movement. What term does the nurse use to describe this type of exercise?

_____

ANSWER: Isometric

Rationale: Quadriceps sets are an isometric exercise involving muscle tension but no change in muscle length or joint movement. Quadriceps sets can reduce weakness and strengthen the muscles used for ambulation.

Nursing process step: Implementation

Client needs category: Physiological integrity

Client needs subcategory: Basic care and comfort

Cognitive level: Comprehension

Basic psychosocial needs

1. The nurse receives a change-of-shift report for a 76-year-old client who had a total hip replacement. The client is not oriented to time, place, or person and is attempting to get out of bed and pull out an I.V. line that's supplying hydration and antibiotics. The client has a vest restraint and bilateral soft wrist restraints. Which of the following actions by the nurse would be appropriate?

Select all that apply:

☐ **A.** Assess and document the behavior that requires continued use of restraints.

☐ **B.** Tie the restraints in quick-release knots.

☐ **C.** Tie the restraints to the side rails of the bed.

☐ **D.** Ask the client if he needs to go to the bathroom and provide range-of-motion exercises every 2 hours.

☐ **E.** Position the vest restraints so that the straps are crossed in the back.

ANSWER: A, B, D

Rationale: The client must be frequently reassessed to determine whether he is ready to have the restraints removed. The information should also be documented. Restraints should be tied in knots that can be released quickly and easily. Toileting and range-of-motion exercises should be performed every 2 hours while a client is in restraints. Restraints should never be secured to side rails because doing so can cause injury if the side rail is lowered without untying the restraint. A vest restraint should be positioned so the straps cross in front of the client, not in the back.

Nursing process step: Implementation

Client needs category: Safe, effective care environment

Client needs subcategory: Safety and infection control

Cognitive level: Application

2. A 62-year-old client has just been diagnosed with terminal cancer and is being transferred to home hospice care. The client's daughter tells the nurse, "I don't know what to say to my mother if she asks me if she's going to die." Which of the following responses by the nurse would be appropriate?

Select all that apply:

☐ **A.** "Don't worry, your mother still has some time left."

☐ **B.** "Let's talk about your mother's illness and how it will progress."

☐ **C.** "You sound like you have some questions about your mother dying. Let's talk about that."

☐ **D.** "Don't worry, hospice will take care of your mother."

☐ **E.** "Tell me how you're feeling about your mother dying."

ANSWER: B, C, E

Rationale: Conveying information and providing clear communication can alleviate fears and strengthen the individual's sense of control. Encouraging verbalization of feelings helps build a therapeutic relationship based on trust and reduces anxiety. Telling the daughter not to worry ignores her feelings and discourages further communication.

Nursing process step: Implementation

Client needs category: Psychosocial integrity

Client needs subcategory: Coping and adaptation

Cognitive level: Analysis

3. While providing care to a 26-year-old married female, the nurse notes multiple ecchymotic areas on her arms and trunk. The color of the ecchymotic areas ranges from blue to purple to yellow. When asked by the nurse how she got these bruises, the client responds, "Oh, I tripped." How should the nurse respond?

Select all that apply:

☐ **A.** Document the client's statement and complete a body map indicating the size, color, shape, location, and type of injuries.

☐ **B.** Report suspicions of abuse to the local authorities.

☐ **C.** Assist the client in developing a safety plan for times of increased violence.

☐ **D.** Call the client's husband to discuss the situation.

☐ **E.** Tell the client that she needs to leave the abusive situation as soon as possible.

☐ **F.** Provide the client with telephone numbers of local shelters and safe houses.

ANSWER: A, C, F

Rationale: The nurse should objectively document her assessment findings. A detailed description of physical findings of abuse in the medical record is essential if legal action is pursued. All women suspected to be victims of abuse should be counseled on a safety plan, which consists of recognizing escalating violence within the family and formulating a plan to exit quickly. The nurse should not report this suspicion of abuse because the client is a competent adult who has the right to self-determination. Nurses do, however, have a duty to report cases of actual or suspected abuse in children or elderly clients. Contacting the client's husband without her consent violates confidentiality. The nurse should respond to the client in a non-threatening manner that promotes trust, rather than ordering her to break off her relationship.

Nursing process step: Implementation

Client needs category: Psychosocial integrity

Client needs subcategory: Psychosocial adaptation

Cognitive level: Analysis

---

4. Elisabeth Kubler-Ross identifies five stages of death and dying. Loss, grief, and intense sadness are symptoms of which stage?

ANSWER: Depression

Rationale: According to Kubler-Ross, the five stages of death and dying are denial and isolation, anger, bargaining, depression, and acceptance. Loss, grief, and intense sadness indicate depression.

Nursing process step: Assessment

Client needs category: Psychosocial integrity

Client needs subcategory: Coping and adaptation

Cognitive level: Application

5. A 26-year-old client with chronic renal failure plans to receive a kidney transplant. Recently, the physician told the client that he is a poor candidate for transplant because of chronic uncontrolled hypertension and diabetes mellitus. Now, the client tells the nurse, "I want to go off dialysis. I'd rather not live than be on this treatment for the rest of my life." Which of the following responses is appropriate?

Select all that apply:

☐ **A.** Take a seat next to the client and sit quietly.

☐ **B.** Say to the client, "We all have days when we don't feel like going on."

☐ **C.** Leave the room to allow the client to collect his thoughts.

☐ **D.** Say to the client, "You're feeling upset about the news you got about the transplant."

☐ **E.** Say to the client, "The treatments are only 3 days a week. You can live with that."

ANSWER: A, D

Rationale: Silence is a therapeutic communication technique that allows the nurse and client to reflect on what has taken place or been said. By waiting quietly and attentively, the nurse encourages the client to initiate and maintain conversation. By reflecting the client's implied feelings, the nurse promotes communication. Using such platitudes as "We all have days when we don't feel like going on" fails to address the client's needs. The nurse should not leave the client alone because he may harm himself. Reminding the client of the treatment frequency doesn't address his feelings.

Nursing process step: Implementation

Client needs category: Psychosocial integrity

Client needs subcategory: Coping and adaptation

Cognitive level: Analysis

6. The nurse is assessing a newly admitted client. When filling out the family assessment, who should the nurse consider to be a part of the client's family?

Select all that apply:

☐ **A.** People related by blood or marriage

☐ **B.** All the people whom the client views as family

☐ **C.** People who live in the same house

☐ **D.** People who the nurse thinks are important to the client

☐ **E.** People who live in the same house with the same racial background as the client

☐ **F.** People who provide for the physical and emotional needs of the client

ANSWER: B, F

Rationale: When providing care to a client, the nurse should consider family members to be all the people whom the client views as family. Family members may also include those people who provide for the physical and emotional needs of the client. The traditional definition of a family has changed and may include people not related by blood or marriage, those of a different racial background, and those who may not live in the same house as the client. Family members are defined by the client, not by the nurse.

Nursing process step: Data collection

Client needs category: Health promotion and maintenance

Client needs subcategory: Growth and development through the life span

Cognitive level: Analysis

7. The nurse is caring for a client whose cultural background is different from her own. Which of the following actions are appropriate?

Select all that apply:

☐ **A.** Consider that nonverbal cues, such as eye contact, may have a different meaning in different cultures.

☐ **B.** Respect the client's cultural beliefs.

☐ **C.** Ask the client if he has cultural or religious requirements that should be considered in his care.

☐ **D.** Explain the nurse's beliefs so that the client will understand the differences.

☐ **E.** Understand that all cultures experience pain in the same way.

ANSWER: A, B, C

Rationale: Nonverbal cues may have different meanings in different cultures. In one culture, eye contact is a sign of disrespect; in another, eye contact shows respect and attentiveness. The nurse should always respect the client's cultural beliefs and ask if he has cultural requirements. This may include food choices or restrictions, body coverings, or time for prayer. The nurse should attempt to understand the client's culture; it is not the client's responsibility to understand the nurse's culture. The nurse should never impose her own beliefs on her clients. Culture influences a client's experience with pain. For example, in one culture pain may be openly expressed whereas in another culture it may be quietly endured.

Nursing process step: Planning

Client needs category: Psychosocial integrity

Client needs subcategory: Coping and adaptation

Cognitive level: Analysis

---

8. The nurse is caring for a 45-year-old married woman who has undergone hemicolectomy for colon cancer. The woman has two children. Which of the following concepts about families should the nurse keep in mind when providing care for this client?

Select all that apply:

☐ **A.** Illness in one family member can affect all members.

☐ **B.** Family roles don't change because of illness.

☐ **C.** A family member may have more than one role at a time in a family.

☐ **D.** Children typically aren't affected by adult illness.

☐ **E.** The effects of an illness on a family depend on the stage of the family's life cycle.

☐ **F.** Changes in sleeping and eating patterns may be signs of stress in a family.

ANSWER: A, C, E, F

Rationale: Illness in one family member can affect all family members, even children. Each member of a family may have several roles to perform. A middle-aged woman, for example, may have the roles of mother, wage-earner, wife, and housekeeper. Families move through certain predictable life cycles (such as birth of a baby, a growing family, adult children leaving home, and grandparenting). The impact of illness on the family may depend on the stage of the life cycle as family members take on different roles and the family structure changes. Illness produces stress in families; changes in eating and sleeping patterns are signs of stress. When one family member can't fulfill a role due to illness, the roles of the other family members are affected.

Nursing process step: Implementation

Client needs category: Health promotion and maintenance

Client needs subcategory: Growth and development through the life span

Cognitive level: Analysis

9. The nurse is performing a nursing assessment on a 72-year-old client admitted with end-stage renal failure. The nurse asks the client if he has a legal document that provides instructions for his care (living will) and names a durable power of attorney for health care if the client cannot act for himself. What is the name of this document?

_____

ANSWER: Advance directive

Rationale: An advance directive is a legal document that's used as a guideline for life-sustaining medical care of a client with an advanced disease or disability who is no longer able to indicate his own wishes. An advance directive includes the living will, which instructs the physician to administer no life-sustaining treatment, and a durable power of attorney for health care, which names another person to act in the client's behalf for medical decisions in the event that the client can't act for himself.

Nursing process step: Assessment

Client needs category: Safe, effective care environment

Client needs subcategory: Management of care

Cognitive level: Comprehension

---

10. A nurse is working with the family of a client who has Alzheimer's disease. The nurse notes that the client's spouse is too exhausted to continue providing care all alone. The adult children live too far away to provide relief on a weekly basis. Which nursing interventions would be most helpful?

Select all that apply:

☐ **A.** Calling a family meeting to tell the absent children that they must participate in helping the client

☐ **B.** Suggesting the spouse seek psychological counseling to help cope with exhaustion

☐ **C.** Recommending community resources for adult day care and respite care

☐ **D.** Encouraging the spouse to talk about the difficulties involved in caring for a loved one with Alzheimer's disease

☐ **E.** Asking whether friends or church members can help with errands or provide short periods of relief

☐ **F.** Recommending that the client be placed in a long-term care facility

ANSWER: C, D, E

Rationale: Many community services exist for Alzheimer's clients and their families. Encouraging use of these resources may make it possible for the client to stay at home and to alleviate the spouse's exhaustion. The nurse can also support the caregiver by urging her to talk about the difficulties she's facing in caring for a spouse. Friends and church members may be able to help provide care to the client, allowing the caregiver time for rest, exercise, or an enjoyable activity. A family meeting to tell the children to participate more would probably be ineffective and may evoke anger or guilt. Counseling may be helpful, but it wouldn't alleviate the caregiver's physical exhaustion and wouldn't address the client's immediate needs. A long-term care facility is not an option until the family is ready to make that decision.

Nursing process step: Implementation

Client needs category: Psychosocial integrity

Client needs subcategory: Coping and adaptation

Cognitive level: Analysis

Medication and I.V. administration

1. A physician prescribes normal saline solution to infuse at a rate of 150 ml/hour for a client admitted with dehydration and pneumonia. How many liters of solution will the client receive during an 8-hour shift?

_____

Rationale: The client is to receive the solution at an infusion rate of 150 ml/hour. 150 ml $\times$ 8 hours = 1,200 ml, the total volume in milliliters the client will receive during an 8-hour shift. Next, convert milliliters to liters by dividing by 1,000. The total volume in liters of normal saline solution that the client will receive in 8 hours is 1.2 L.

Nursing process step: Planning

Client needs category: Physiological integrity

Client needs subcategory: Pharmacological and parenteral therapies

Cognitive level: Analysis

2. A client is prescribed heparin 6,000 U subcutaneously every 12 hours for deep vein thrombosis prophylaxis. The pharmacy dispenses a vial containing 10,000 U/ml. How many milliliters of heparin should the nurse administer?

_____

ANSWER: 0.6

Rationale: The following formula is used to calculate drug dosages:

Dose on hand/Quantity on hand = Dose desired/X

The dose dispensed by the pharmacy is 10,000 U/1 ml and the desired dose is 6,000 U. The nurse should use the following equations:

$$10,000 \text{ U}/1 \text{ ml} = 6,000 \text{ U}/X$$

$$10,000 \text{ U } (X) = 6,000 \text{ U (ml)}$$

$$X = 6,000 \text{ U (ml)}/10,000 \text{ U}$$

$$X = 0.6 \text{ ml}$$

Nursing process step: Planning

Client needs category: Physiological integrity

Client needs subcategory: Pharmacological and parenteral therapies

Cognitive level: Analysis

3. A client admitted to the hospital with diabetic ketoacidosis is receiving a continuous infusion of regular insulin. The physician orders an I.V. containing dextrose 5% in water to be started when the client's blood glucose level reaches 250 mg/dl. This is known as what type of I.V. solution?

_____

ANSWER: Isotonic

Rationale: Dextrose 5% in water is an isotonic solution. A solution is isotonic if its osmolarity falls within or near the normal range for serum osmolarity (240 to 340 mOsm/L). The osmolarity of dextrose 5% in water is 260 mOsm/L.

Nursing process step: Implementation

Client needs category: Physiological integrity

Client needs subcategory: Pharmacological and parenteral therapies

Cognitive level: Comprehension

---

4. The cardiologist prescribes digoxin (Lanoxin) 125 µg by mouth every morning for a client diagnosed with heart failure. The pharmacy dispenses tablets that contain 0.25 mg each. How many tablets should the nurse administer in each dose?

_____

ANSWER: ½

Rationale: The nurse should begin by converting 125 µg to milligrams:

$$125 \text{ µg}/1,000 = 0.125 \text{ mg.}$$

The following formula is used to calculate drug dosages:

Dose on hand/Quantity on hand = Dose desired/X

The nurse should use the following equations:

$$0.25 \text{ mg}/1 = 0.125 \text{ mg}/1 \text{ tablet}$$

$$0.25X = 0.125$$

$$X = 0.5 \text{ tablet}$$

Nursing process step: Implementation

Client needs category: Physiological integrity

Client needs subcategory: Pharmacological and parenteral therapies

Cognitive level: Analysis

5. A 75-year-old client is admitted to the hospital with lower G.I. bleeding. His hemoglobin on admission to the emergency department is 7.3 g/dl. The physician prescribes 2 U of packed red blood cells to infuse over 1 hour each. The blood administration set has a drip factor of 10 gtt/ml. What is the flow rate in drops per minute?

_____

Rationale: Each unit of packed red blood cells contains 250 ml. Each unit is to infuse over 1 hour (60 minutes).

Use the following equation:

$$250 \text{ ml}/60 \text{ minutes} = 4.16 \text{ ml.}$$

Multiply by the drip factor:

$$4.16 \text{ ml} \times 10 \text{ gtt} = 41.6 \text{ gtt/minute (42 gtt/minute).}$$

Nursing process step: Implementation

Client needs category: Physiological integrity

Client needs subcategory: Pharmacological and parenteral therapies

Cognitive level: Analysis

---

6. The nurse is preparing a teaching plan for a client who was prescribed enalapril maleate (Vasotec) for treatment of hypertension. Which of the following should the nurse include in the teaching plan?

Select all that apply:

☐ **A.** Tell the client to avoid salt substitutions.

☐ **B.** Tell the client that light-headedness is a common adverse effect that need not be reported.

☐ **C.** Inform the client that he may have a sore throat for the first few days of therapy.

☐ **D.** Advise the client to report facial swelling or difficulty breathing immediately.

☐ **E.** Tell the client that blood tests will be necessary every 3 weeks for 2 months and periodically after that.

☐ **F.** Advise the client not to change position suddenly to minimize orthostatic hypotension.

ANSWER: A, D, F

Rationale: When teaching the client about enalapril maleate, the nurse should tell him to avoid salt substitutions, as these products may contain potassium that can cause light-headedness and syncope. Facial swelling or difficulty breathing should be reported immediately; the drug may cause angioedema, which would require discontinuation of the drug. The client should also be advised to change position slowly to minimize orthostatic hypotension. The nurse should tell the client to report light-headedness, especially in the first few days of therapy, so dosage adjustments can be made. The client should report signs of infection, such as sore throat and fever, because the drug may decrease the white blood cell count. White blood cell and differential counts should be performed before treatment, every 2 weeks for 3 months, and periodically thereafter.

Nursing process step: Planning

Client needs category: Physiological integrity

Client needs subcategory: Pharmacological and parenteral therapies

Cognitive level: Application

7. After sustaining a closed head injury, a client is prescribed phenytoin (Dilantin) 100 mg I.V. every 8 hours for seizure prophylaxis. Which nursing interventions are necessary when administering phenytoin?

Select all that apply:

☐ **A.** Administer phenytoin through any peripheral I.V. site.

☐ **B.** Mix I.V. doses in mixtures containing dextrose 5% in water.

☐ **C.** Administer an I.V. bolus no faster than 50 mg/minute.

☐ **D.** Monitor ECG, blood pressure, and respiratory status continuously when administering phenytoin I.V.

☐ **E.** Don't use an inline filter when administering the drug.

☐ **F.** Know that early toxicity may cause drowsiness, nausea, vomiting, nystagmus, ataxia, dysarthria, tremor, and slurred speech.

ANSWER: C, D, F

Rationale: If using I.V. bolus, administer by slow (50 mg/minute) I.V. push; too rapid of an injection may cause hypotension and circulatory collapse. Continuous monitoring of ECG, blood pressure, and respiratory status is essential when administering phenytoin I.V. Early toxicity may cause drowsiness, nausea, vomiting, nystagmus, ataxia, dysarthria, tremor, and slurred speech. Later, hypotension, arrhythmias, respiratory depression, and coma may occur. Death is caused by respiratory and circulatory depression. Phenytoin shouldn't be administered by I.V. push in veins on the back of the hand; larger veins are needed to prevent discoloration associated with purple glove syndrome. Mix I.V. doses in normal saline solution and use within 30 minutes; mixtures with dextrose 5% in water will precipitate. Use of an inline filter is recommended.

Nursing process step: Implementation

Client needs category: Physiological integrity

Client needs subcategory: Pharmacological and parenteral therapies

Cognitive level: Application

---

8. A 53-year-old client returns to his room from the postanesthesia care unit after undergoing right hemicolectomy. The physician orders 1 L of dextrose 5% in half-normal saline solution to infuse at 125 ml/hour. The drip factor of the available I.V. tubing is 15 gtt/ml. What is the drip rate in drops per minute?

_____

ANSWER: 31

Rationale: The flow rate is 125 ml/hour or 125 ml/60 minutes. Use the following equation:

Drip rate = 125 ml/60 minutes × 15 gtt/1 ml.

The drip rate is 31.25 gtt/minute (31 gtt/minute).

Nursing process step: Implementation

Client needs category: Physiological integrity

Client needs subcategory: Pharmacological and parenteral therapies

Cognitive level: Application

9. The physician prescribes heparin 25,000 U in 250 ml of normal saline solution to infuse at 600 U/hour for a client who suffered an acute myocardial infarction. After 6 hours of heparin therapy, the client's partial thromboplastin time is subtherapeutic. The physician orders an increase in the infusion to 800 U/hour. The nurse should set the infusion pump to deliver how many milliliters per hour?

_____

ANSWER: 8

Rationales: The following formula is used to calculate drug dosages:

Dose on hand/Quantity on hand = Dose desired/X

The nurse should use the following equations:

25,000 U/250 ml = 800 U/hour/X.

Cross-multiply to solve for X and divide each side of the equation by 25,000 U;

X = 8 ml/hour.

Nursing process step: Implementation

Client needs category: Physiological integrity

Client needs subcategory: Pharmacological and parenteral therapies

Cognitive level: Application

---

10. After undergoing small-bowel resection, a client is prescribed metronidazole (Flagyl) 500 mg I.V. The mixed I.V. solution contains 100 ml. The nurse is to run the drug over 30 minutes. The drip factor of the available I.V. tubing is 15 gtt/ml. What is the drip rate?

_____

ANSWER: 50

Rationale: Use the following equation:

100 ml/30 minutes $\times$ 15 gtt/1 ml = 49.9 gtt/minute (50 gtt/minute)

Nursing process step: Implementation

Client needs category: Physiological integrity

Client needs subcategory: Pharmacological and parenteral therapies

Cognitive level: Application

11. A client with acute renal failure is prescribed regular insulin 10 U I.V. along with 50 ml of dextrose 50%. What electrolyte imbalance is this client most likely experiencing?

_____

ANSWER: Hyperkalemia

Rationale: Regular insulin I.V. administered concomitantly with 50 ml of dextrose 50% helps shift potassium from the extracellular fluid into the cell, which normalizes serum potassium levels in the client with hyperkalemia.

Nursing process step: Implementation

Client needs category: Physiological integrity

Client needs subcategory: Physiological adaptation

Cognitive level: Analysis

_____

12. After suffering an acute myocardial infarction, a client with a history of type 1 diabetes is prescribed metoprolol (Lopressor) I.V. Which nursing interventions are associated with I.V. metoprolol administration?

Select all that apply:

☐ **A.** Monitor glucose levels closely.

☐ **B.** Monitor for heart block and bradycardia.

☐ **C.** Monitor blood pressure closely.

☐ **D.** Mix the drug in 50 ml of dextrose 5% in water and infuse over 30 minutes.

☐ **E.** Know that the drug isn't compatible with morphine.

ANSWER: A, B, C

Rationale: Metoprolol masks the common signs of hypoglycemia; therefore, glucose levels should be monitored closely in diabetics. Monitor the client for the development of heart block or bradycardia. When used to treat an MI, metoprolol is contraindicated in clients with heart rates less than 45 beats/minute and any degree of heart block. Monitor blood pressure frequently; metoprolol masks common signs and symptoms of shock, such as decreased blood pressure. Give the drug undiluted by direct injection. Although mixing with other drugs should be avoided, studies have shown metoprolol is compatible when mixed with meperidine hydrochloride or morphine sulfate, or when administered with alteplase infusion at a Y-site connection.

Nursing process step: Implementation

Client needs category: Physiological integrity

Client needs subcategory: Pharmacological and parenteral therapies

Cognitive level: Application

1. A client who was involved in a motor vehicle accident is admitted to the intensive care unit. The emergency department admission record indicates that the client hit her head on the steering wheel. The client complains of a headache and a nursing assessment reveals that she has difficulty comprehending language and diminished hearing. Based on these findings, the nurse suspects injury to which lobe of the brain?

ANSWER: Temporal

Rationale: The temporal lobe controls hearing, language comprehension, and the storage and recall of memories.

Nursing process step: Assessment

Client needs category: Physiological integrity

Client needs subcategory: Physiological adaptation

Cognitive level: Analysis

2. The nurse is assessing a client who reports burning on urination and a low-grade fever. On physical examination, the nurse notes right-sided costovertebral tenderness. Identify the area the nurse percussed to elicit this sign.

ANSWER:

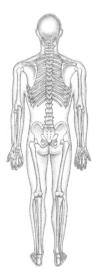

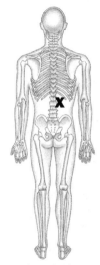

Rationale: To determine whether costovertebral tenderness (a sign of glomerulonephritis) is present, the nurse should percuss the costovertebral angle (the angle over each kidney that's formed by the lateral and downward curve of the lowest rib and the vertebral column). The costovertebral angle can be percussed by placing the palm of one hand over the costovertebral angle and striking it with the fist of the other hand.

Nursing process step: Assessment

Client needs category: Physiological integrity

Client needs subcategory: Physiological adaptation

Cognitive level: Application

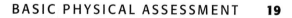

3. The nurse is assessing a client's abdomen. Identify the area where the nurse's hand should be placed to palpate the liver.

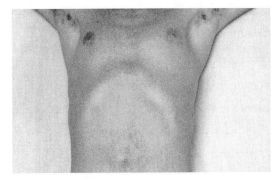

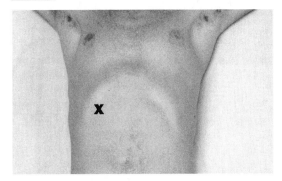

Rationale: The nurse can best palpate the liver by standing on the client's right side and placing her right hand on the client's abdomen, to the right of midline. She should point the fingers of her right hand toward the client's head, just under the right rib margin.

Nursing process step: Assessment

Client needs category: Health promotion and maintenance

Client needs subcategory: Prevention and early detection of disease

Cognitive level: Application

---

4. While examining the hands of a client with osteoarthritis, the nurse notes Heberden's nodes on the second (pointer) finger. Identify the area on the finger where the nurse observed the node.

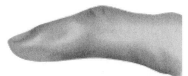

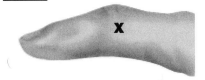

Rationale: Heberden's nodes appear on the distal interphalangeal joints. These bony and cartilaginous enlargements are usually hard and painless and typically occur in middle-aged and elderly clients with osteoarthritis.

Nursing process step: Assessment

Client needs category: Physiological integrity

Client needs subcategory: Physiological adaptation

Cognitive level: Application

5. The nurse is percussing the client's abdomen. Identify the area where liver dullness is best percussed.

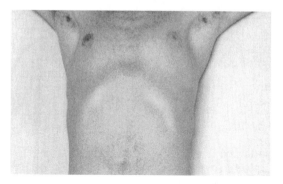

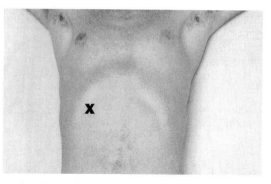

Rationale: Liver dullness is best heard over the right anterior lower rib cage. To hear this, the nurse should percuss the abdomen in the right midclavicular line, starting at a level below the umbilicus (in an area of tympany, not dullness). She should then percuss upward toward the liver.

Nursing process step: Assessment

Client needs category: Health promotion and maintenance

Client needs subcategory: Prevention and early detection of disease

Cognitive level: Application

---

6. A 60-year old client reports to the nurse that he has a rash on his back and right flank. The nurse observes elevated, round, blisterlike lesions that are filled with clear fluid. When documenting the findings, what medical term should the nurse use to describe these lesions?

ANSWER: Vesicles

Rationale: Vesicles are raised, round, serous-filled lesions that are usually less than 1 cm in diameter. Examples of vesicles include chickenpox (varicella) and shingles (herpes zoster).

Nursing process step: Assessment

Client needs category: Health promotion and maintenance

Client needs subcategory: Prevention and early detection of disease

Cognitive level: Comprehension

7. An elderly client has a history of aortic stenosis. Identify the area where the nurse should place the stethoscope to best hear the murmur.

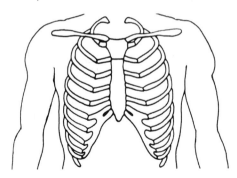

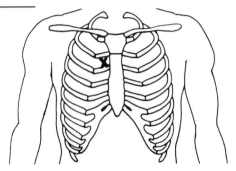

Rationale: The murmur of aortic stenosis is low-pitched, rough, and rasping. It is heard loudest in the second intercostal space to the right of the sternum.

Nursing process step: Assessment

Client needs category: Physiological integrity

Client needs subcategory: Physiological adaptation

Cognitive level: Application

---

8. The nurse is assessing a client who has a rash on his chest and upper arms. Which questions should the nurse ask in order to gain further information about the client's rash?

Select all that apply:

☐ **A.** "When did the rash start?"

☐ **B.** "Are you allergic to any medications, foods, or pollen?"

☐ **C.** "How old are you?"

☐ **D.** "What have you been using to treat the rash?"

☐ **E.** "Have you recently traveled outside the country?"

☐ **F.** "Do you smoke cigarettes or drink alcohol?"

ANSWER: A, B, D, E

Rationale: When assessing a client who has a rash, the nurse should first find out when the rash began; this information can identify where the rash is in the disease process and assists with the correct diagnosis. The nurse should also ask about allergies because rashes related to allergies can occur when a person changes medications, eats new foods, or comes into contact with agents in the air, such as pollen. It's also important for the nurse to find out how the client has been treating the rash because treating the rash with topical ointments or taking oral medications may make the rash worse. The nurse should ask about recent travel because travel outside the country exposes the client to foreign foods and environments, which can contribute to the onset of a rash. Although the client's age and smoking and drinking habits can be important to know, this information will not provide further insight to the rash or its cause.

Nursing process step: Assessment

Client needs category: Physiological integrity

Client needs subcategory: Physiological adaptation

Cognitive level: Application

---

9. While assessing a client's spine for abnormal curvatures, the nurse notes lordosis. Identify the area of the spine that is affected by lordosis.

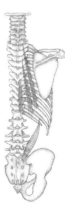

ANSWER:

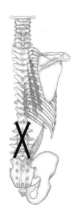

Rationale: Lordosis is characterized by an accentuated curve of the lumbar area of the spine.

Nursing process step: Assessment

Client needs category: Health promotion and maintenance

Client needs subcategory: Prevention and early detection of disease

Cognitive level: Application

---

10. The nurse is auscultating a client's lungs. Identify the area on the client's vertebrae, representing the base of the lungs, where the nurse expects the breath sounds to end at end expiration.

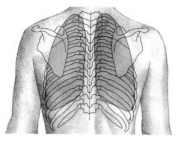

ANSWER:

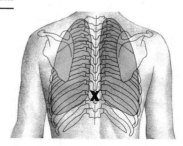

Rationale: Using posterior landmarks, the lungs extend from the cervical area to the level of the 10th thoracic vertebrae (T10) at the end of expiration.

Nursing process step: Assessment

Client needs category: Health promotion and maintenance

Client needs subcategory: Prevention and early detection of disease

Cognitive level: Application

11. The nurse is performing an otoscopic examination of a client with ear pain. The nurse notes that the tympanic membrane is bulging and red. Identify the structure that the nurse is assessing.

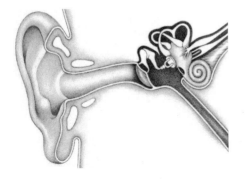

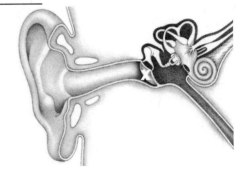

Rationale: The tympanic membrane separates the external and middle ear and may appear red and bulging in a client with otitis media.

Nursing process step: Assessment

Client needs category: Physiological integrity

Client needs subcategory: Physiological adaptation

Cognitive level: Application

---

12. The nurse is performing a cardiac assessment on a client with a suspected murmur. Identify the area where the nurse should place the stethoscope to auscultate the area referred to as Erb's point.

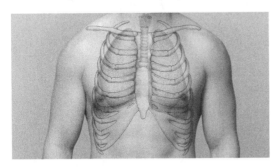

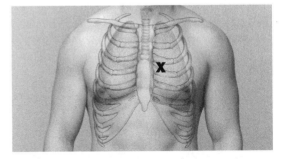

Rationale: Erb's point is located at the third left intercostal space, close to the sternum. Murmurs of both aortic and pulmonic origin may be heard at Erb's point.

Nursing process step: Assessment

Client needs category: Health promotion and maintenance

Client needs subcategory: Prevention and early detection of disease

Cognitive level: Application

13. The nurse is performing a head and neck assessment on a client who reports fatigue. Identify the area that the nurse palpates to assess the occipital lymph nodes of the head.

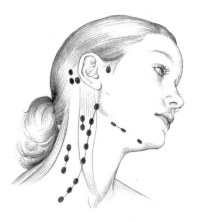

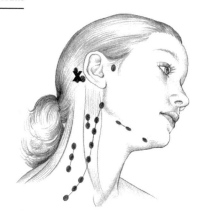

Rationale: Using the pads of the fingers, the nurse bilaterally palpates the area behind the ears to assess the occipital lymph nodes.

Nursing process step: Assessment

Client needs category: Physiological integrity

Client needs subcategory: Physiological adaptation

Cognitive level: Application

---

14. The nurse is performing a cardiac assessment. Identify where the nurse places the stethoscope to best auscultate the pulmonic valve.

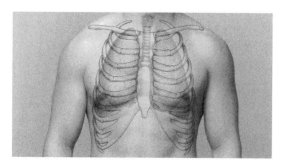

ANSWER:

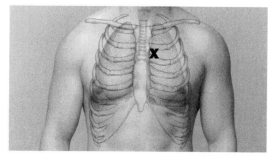

Rationale: The pulmonic area is best heard at the second intercostal space, just left of the sternum.

Nursing process step: Assessment

Client needs category: Health promotion and maintenance

Client needs subcategory: Prevention and early detection of disease

Cognitive level: Application

Part 2

Medical-surgical nursing

1. A septic client with hypotension is being treated with dopamine hydrochloride (Inotropin). The nurse asks a colleague to double-check the dosage that the client is receiving. There are 400 mg of dopamine hydrochloride (Inotropin) in 250 ml, the infusion pump is running at 23 ml/hour, and the client weighs 79.5 kg. How many micrograms per kilogram per minute is the client receiving?

_____

ANSWER: 7.71

Rationale: First, calculate how many micrograms per milliliter of dopamine hydrochloride (Inotropin) are in the bag: 400 mg/250 ml = 1.6 mg/ml

Next, convert milligrams to micrograms:

1.6 mg/ml × 1,000 mcg/mg = 1,600 mcg/ml

Lastly, calculate the dose:

1,600 mcg/ml × 23 ml/hour/79.5 kg

79.5 kg/60 minutes/hour = 7.71 mcg/kg/minute

Nursing process step: Analysis

Client needs category: Physiological integrity

Client needs subcategory: Pharmacological and parenteral therapies

Cognitive level: Analysis

---

2. A client with deep vein thrombosis has an I.V. infusion of heparin sodium infusing at 1,500 U/hour. The concentration in the bag is 25,000 U/500 ml. How much should the nurse document as intake from this infusion for an 8-hour shift?

_____

ANSWER: 240

Rationale: First, calculate how many units are in each milliliter of the medication:

25,000 U/500 ml = 50 U/ml

Next, calculate how many milliliters the client receives each hour:

1 ml/50 U × 1,500 U/hour = 30 ml/hour

Lastly, multiply by 8 hours:

30 ml/hour × 8 hours = 240 ml

Nursing process step: Analysis

Client needs category: Physiological integrity

Client needs subcategory: Pharmacological and parenteral therapies

Cognitive level: Analysis

3. The nurse is evaluating the following telemetry strip from one of her clients. What arrhythmia should the nurse document?

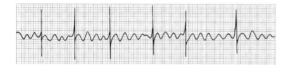

_____

4. The nurse is interpreting a client's telemetry strip. If the QT interval is 0.52 second and the R-R interval is 1.72 seconds, how many seconds is the QTc interval (the QT interval corrected for the heart rate)?

_____

ANSWER: Atrial flutter

Rationale: Characteristics of atrial flutter include the presence of flutter waves, a regular atrial rhythm, a rapid atrial rate, an immeasurable PR interval, and a regular or irregular ventricular rhythm (in this case, irregular).

Nursing process step: Analysis

Client needs category: Physiological integrity

Client needs subcategory: Physiological adaptation

Cognitive level: Analysis

ANSWER: 0.39

Rationale: To correct the QT interval for variations in heart rate, divide the measured QT interval by the square root of the measured R-R interval.

$$\text{Square root of } 1.72 = 1.31$$

$$0.52 \div 1.31 = 0.39 \text{ second}$$

The QTc should be less than 0.44 seconds in men, and less than 0.46 seconds in women.

Nursing process step: Analysis

Client needs category: Physiological integrity

Client needs subcategory: Reduction of risk potential

Cognitive level: Application

5. A 32-year-old female with systemic lupus erythematosus (SLE) complains that her hands become pale, blue, and painful when exposed to the cold. What disorder should the nurse cite as an explanation for these sign and symptoms?

_____

ANSWER: Raynaud's disease

Rationale: Raynaud's disease results from reduced blood flow to the extremities when exposed to cold or stress. It's commonly associated with connective tissue disorders such as SLE. Signs and symptoms include pallor, coldness, numbness, throbbing pain, and cyanosis.

Nursing process step: Implementation

Client needs category: Physiological integrity

Client needs subcategory: Physiological adaptation

Cognitive level: Application

---

6. A client with a bicuspid aortic valve has severe stenosis and is scheduled for valve replacement. While teaching the client about his condition and upcoming surgery, the nurse shows him a heart illustration. Identify the valve that the nurse should indicate will be replaced.

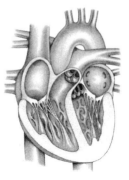

ANSWER:

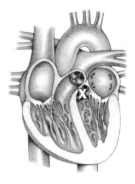

Rationale: The aortic valve is located between the left ventricle and the aorta. It's one of the semilunar valves and normally has three cusps. A person with a bicuspid aortic valve is at risk for aortic stenosis and aortic regurgitation. This impaired blood flow through the valve leads to increased pumping pressure of the left ventricle.

Nursing process step: Planning

Client needs category: Physiological integrity

Client needs subcategory: Physiological adaptation

Cognitive level: Application

7. The nurse is evaluating the 12-lead electrocardiogram (ECG) of a client experiencing an inferior wall myocardial infarction (MI). While conferring with the team, she correctly identifies which of the following ECG changes associated with an evolving MI?

Select all that apply:

☐ **A.** Notched T-wave

☐ **B.** Presence of a U-wave

☐ **C.** T-wave inversion

☐ **D.** Prolonged PR-interval

☐ **E.** ST-segment elevation

☐ **F.** Pathologic Q-wave

ANSWER: C, E, F

Rationale: T-wave inversion, ST-segment elevation, and a pathologic Q-wave are all signs of tissue hypoxia which occur during an MI. Ischemia results from inadequate blood supply to the myocardial tissue and is reflected by T-wave inversion. Injury results from prolonged ischemia and is reflected by ST-segment elevation. Q-waves may become evident when the injury progresses to infarction. A notched T-wave may indicate pericarditis in an adult client. The presence of a U-wave may or may not be apparent on a normal ECG; it represents repolarization of the Purkinje fibers. A prolonged PR-interval is associated with first-degree atrioventricular block.

Nursing process step: Evaluation

Client needs category: Physiological integrity

Client needs subcategory: Physiological adaptation

Cognitive level: Analysis

---

8. The nurse is awaiting the arrival of a client from the emergency department who is being admitted with a left ventricular myocardial infarction. In caring for this client, the nurse should be alert for which of the following signs and symptoms of left-sided heart failure?

Select all that apply:

☐ **A.** Jugular venous distention

☐ **B.** Hepatomegaly

☐ **C.** Dyspnea

☐ **D.** Crackles

☐ **E.** Tachycardia

☐ **F.** Right upper quadrant pain

ANSWER: C, D, E

Rationale: Signs and symptoms of left-sided heart failure include dyspnea, orthopnea, and paroxysmal nocturnal dyspnea; fatigue; nonproductive cough and crackles; hemoptysis; point of maximal impulse displaced toward the left anterior axillary line; tachycardia and S3 and S4 heart sounds; and cool, pale skin. Jugular venous distention, hepatomegaly, and right upper quadrant pain are all signs of right-sided heart failure.

Nursing process step: Assessment

Client needs category: Physiological integrity

Client needs subcategory: Physiological adaptation

Cognitive level: Application

9. A client is admitted to the emergency department after complaining of acute chest pain radiating down his left arm. Which of the following laboratory studies would be indicated?

Select all that apply:

☐ **A.** Hemoglobin and hematocrit

☐ **B.** Serum glucose

☐ **C.** Creatinine phosphokinase (CPK)

☐ **D.** Troponin T and troponin I

☐ **E.** Myoglobin

☐ **F.** Blood urea nitrogen (BUN)

ANSWER: C, D, E

Rationale: Levels of CPK, troponin T, and troponin I elevate because of cellular damage. Myoglobin elevation is an early indicator of myocardial damage. Hemoglobin, hematocrit, serum glucose, and BUN levels don't provide information related to myocardial ischemia.

Nursing process step: Planning

Client needs category: Health promotion and maintenance

Client needs subcategory: Prevention and early detection of disease

Cognitive level: Application

---

10. A client is prescribed lisinopril (Zestril) for treatment of hypertension. He asks the nurse about possible adverse effects. The nurse should teach him about which of the following common adverse effects of ACE inhibitors?

Select all that apply:

☐ **A.** Constipation

☐ **B.** Dizziness

☐ **C.** Headache

☐ **D.** Hyperglycemia

☐ **E.** Hypotension

☐ **F.** Impotence

ANSWER: B, C, E

Rationale: Dizziness, headache, and hypotension are all common adverse effects of lisinopril and other ACE inhibitors. Lisinopril may cause diarrhea, not constipation. Lisinopril isn't known to cause hyperglycemia or impotence.

Nursing process step: Implementation

Client needs category: Physiological integrity

Client needs subcategory: Pharmacological and parenteral therapies

Cognitive level: Application

11. The nurse is performing a 12-lead electrocardio-gram (ECG) on a client who's complaining of chest pain. Identify the area where lead V_6 should be placed.

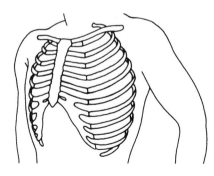

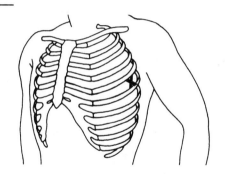

Rationale: The V_6 lead is placed at the 5th intercostal space at the midaxillary line. Correct placement of the leads is essential when performing a 12-lead ECG to accurately document the electrical potential of the heart. V_6 is one of the precordial leads and, in combination with the other leads, records potential in the horizontal plane.

Nursing process step: Implementation

Client needs category: Physiological integrity

Client needs subcategory: Reduction of risk potential

Cognitive level: Application

---

12. The nurse is counseling a 52-year-old client about risk factors for hypertension. Which of the following should the nurse list as risk factors for *primary* hypertension?

Select all that apply:

☐ **A.** Obesity

☐ **B.** Diabetes mellitus

☐ **C.** Head injury

☐ **D.** Stress

☐ **E.** Oral contraceptives

☐ **F.** High intake of sodium or saturated fat

ANSWER: A, D, F

Rationale: Obesity, stress, high intake of sodium or saturated fat, and family history are all risk factors for primary hypertension. Diabetes mellitus, head injury, and oral contraceptives are risk factors for secondary hypertension.

Nursing process step: Assessment

Client needs category: Health promotion and maintenance

Client needs subcategory: Prevention and early detection of disease

Cognitive level: Application

13. The nurse is caring for a client with first-degree atrioventricular (AV) block. Identify the area in the conduction cycle of the heart where this block occurs.

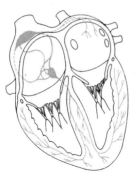

ANSWER:

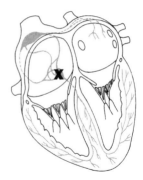

Rationale: First-degree AV block is a conduction disturbance in which electrical impulses flow normally from the sinoatrial (SA) node through the atria, but are delayed at the AV node.

Nursing process step: Assessment

Client needs category: Physiological integrity

Client needs subcategory: Physiological adaptation

Cognitive level: Analysis

Oncologic disorders

1. A client is in the terminal stage of cancer and he's being transferred to hospice care. Which information should the nurse include in the teaching plan regarding hospice care?

Select all that apply:

- ☐ **A.** Focus of care is on control of symptoms and relief of pain.

- ☐ **B.** A multidisciplinary team provides care.

- ☐ **C.** Services are provided on the ability to pay.

- ☐ **D.** Hospice care is provided only in hospice centers.

- ☐ **E.** Bereavement care is provided to the family.

- ☐ **F.** Care is provided in the home, independent of physicians.

ANSWER: A, B, E

Rationale: Hospice care focuses on the control of symptoms and the relief of pain at the end of life. A multidisciplinary team — possibly consisting of nurses, physicians, chaplains, aides, and volunteers — provides the care. After the client's death, hospice provides bereavement care to the grieving family. Hospice services are provided based on need, not on the ability to pay. Hospice care may be provided in a variety of settings, such as freestanding hospice centers, at home, in a hospital, or in a long-term care facility. Care is provided under the direction of a physician, who's a key member of the care team.

Nursing process step: Planning

Client needs category: Physiological integrity

Client needs subcategory: Basic care and comfort

Cognitive level: Application

2. An adult client with Hodgkin's disease who weighs 143 lb is to receive vincristine (Oncovin) 25 mcg/kg I.V. What is the correct dose in micrograms that the client should receive?

_____

ANSWER: 1,625

Rationale: First, convert the client's weight from pounds to kilograms:

$$1 \text{ lb} = 2.2 \text{ kg};$$

$$143 \text{ lb} = X \text{ kg};$$

$$143 \text{ lb}/2.2 \text{ kg} = 65 \text{ kg}.$$

Next, multiply the weight in kilograms by the number of micrograms desired per kilogram:

$$65 \text{ kg} \times 25 \text{ mcg} = 1,625 \text{ mcg}$$

Nursing process step: Implementation

Client needs category: Physiological integrity

Client needs subcategory: Pharmacological and parenteral therapies

Cognitive level: Application

3. What diagnostic study is it recommended that all women older than age 50 receive annually?

_____

ANSWER: Mammography

Rationale: In order to detect a breast tumor early, the National Cancer Institute and the American Cancer Society recommend annual mammography for women older than age 50.

Nursing process step: Planning

Client needs category: Health promotion and maintenance

Client needs subcategory: Prevention and early detection of disease

Cognitive level: Knowledge

4. A client with laryngeal cancer has undergone laryngectomy and is now receiving radiation therapy to the head and neck. The nurse should monitor the client for which of the following adverse effects of external radiation?

Select all that apply:

☐ **A.** Xerostomia

☐ **B.** Stomatitis

☐ **C.** Thrombocytopenia

☐ **D.** Cystitis

☐ **E.** Dysgeusia

☐ **F.** Leukopenia

ANSWER: A, B, E

Rationale: Radiation of the head and neck often produces dry mouth (xerostomia), irritation of the oral mucus membranes (stomatitis), and diminished sense of taste (dysgeusia). Thrombocytopenia (reduced platelet count) and leukopenia (reduced white blood cell count) may occur with systemic radiation; cystitis may occur with radiation of the genitourinary system.

Nursing process step: Assessment

Client needs category: Physiological integrity

Client needs subcategory: Reduction of risk potential

Cognitive level: Application

---

5. A client with bladder cancer undergoes surgical removal of the bladder with construction of an ileal conduit. What assessments by the nurse indicate that the client is developing complications?

Select all that apply:

☐ **A.** Urine output greater than 30 ml/hr

☐ **B.** Dusky appearance of the stoma

☐ **C.** Stoma protrusion from the skin

☐ **D.** Mucus shreds in the urine collection bag

☐ **E.** Edema of the stoma during the first 24 hours after surgery

☐ **F.** Sharp abdominal pain with rigidity

ANSWER: B, C, F

Rationale: A dusky appearance of the stoma indicates decreased blood supply; a healthy stoma should appear beefy-red. Protrusion indicates prolapse of the stoma and sharp abdominal pain with rigidity suggests peritonitis. A urinary output greater than 30 ml/hr is a sign of adequate renal perfusion and is a normal finding. Because mucous membranes are used to create the conduit, mucous in the urine is expected. Stomal edema is a normal finding during the first 24 hours after surgery.

Nursing process step: Assessment

Client needs category: Physiological integrity

Client needs subcategory: Reduction of risk potential

Cognitive level: Analysis

6. A client who is receiving chemotherapy for breast cancer develops myelosuppression. Which of the following instructions should the nurse include in the client's discharge teaching plan?

Select all that apply:

☐ **A.** Avoid people who have recently received attenuated vaccines.

☐ **B.** Avoid activities that may cause bleeding.

☐ **C.** Wash hands frequently.

☐ **D.** Increase intake of fresh fruits and vegetables.

☐ **E.** Avoid crowded places such as shopping malls.

☐ **F.** Treat a sore throat with over-the-counter products.

ANSWER: A, B, C, E

Rationale: Chemotherapy can cause myelosuppression, which is reduced numbers of red blood cells, white blood cells, and platelets. A client receiving chemotherapy needs to avoid people who have been vaccinated recently because an exaggerated reaction may occur. Because platelet counts are reduced, the client also needs to avoid activities that could cause trauma and bleeding. The client should wash her hands frequently because hand washing is the best way to prevent the spread of infection. A client receiving chemotherapy should avoid crowded places, as well as people with colds during the flu season, because she has a reduced ability to fight infection. Fresh fruits and vegetables should be avoided because they can harbor bacteria that can't be removed easily by washing. Signs and symptoms of infection, such as a sore throat, fever, and a cough, should be reported immediately to the physician.

Nursing process step: Planning

Client needs category: Physiological integrity

Client needs subcategory: Reduction of risk potential

Cognitive level: Application

7. Following lobectomy for lung cancer, a client receives a chest tube connected to a three-chamber chest drainage system. The nurse observes that the drainage system is functioning correctly when she notes tidal movements or fluctuations in which compartment of the system as the client breathes?

ANSWER: Water-seal

Rationale: Fluctuations in the water-seal compartment are called tidal movements and indicate normal function of the system as the pressure in the tubing changes with the client's respirations.

Nursing process step: Assessment

Client needs category: Physiological integrity

Client needs subcategory: Reduction of risk potential

Cognitive level: Application

8. After receiving chemotherapy for lung cancer, a client's platelet count falls to 98,000/μl. What term should the nurse use to describe this low platelet count?

_____

ANSWER: Thrombocytopenia

Rationale: A normal platelet count is 140,000 to 400,000/μl in adults. Chemotherapeutic agents produce bone marrow depression, resulting in reduced red blood cell counts (anemia), reduced white blood cell counts (leukopenia), and reduced platelet counts (thrombocytopenia).

Nursing process step: Implementation

Client needs category: Physiological integrity

Client needs subcategory: Physiological adaptation

Cognitive level: Comprehension

Gastrointestinal disorders

1. The nurse is reviewing the causes of gastroesophageal reflux disease (GERD) with a client. What area of the GI tract should the nurse identify as the cause of reduced pressure associated with GERD?

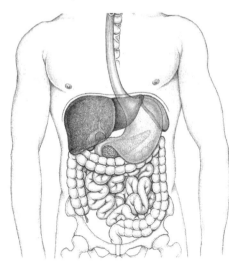

ANSWER:

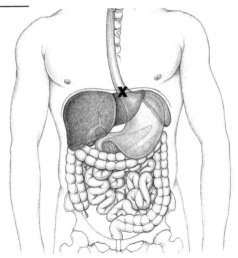

Rationale: Normally, there is enough pressure around the lower esophageal sphincter (LES) to close it. Reflux occurs when LES pressure is deficient or when pressure in the stomach exceeds LES pressure.

Nursing process step: Implementation

Client needs category: Health promotion and maintenance

Client needs subcategory: Prevention and early detection of disease

Cognitive level: Application

2. A 78-year-old client with pancreatic cancer has the following blood chemistry profile:

Glucose, fasting: 204 mg/dL
BUN: 12 mg/dL
Creatinine: 0.9 mg/dL
Sodium: 136 mEq/L
Potassium: 2.2 mEq/L
Chloride: 99 mEq/L
CO_2: 33 mEq/L

Which of these results should the nurse identify as critical and report immediately?

_____

ANSWER: Potassium

Rationale: A normal potassium level is 3.8 to 5.5mEq/L. Severe hypokalemia can cause cardiac and respiratory arrest, possibly leading to death. Hypokalemia also depresses the release of insulin and results in glucose intolerance. The glucose level is above normal (normal is 75 to 110 mg/dL) and the chloride level is a bit low (normal is 100 to 110 mEq/L). However, while these levels should be reported, neither is life-threatening. The BUN (normal is 8 to 26 mg/dL) and creatinine (normal is 0.8 to 1.4 mg/dL) are within normal range.

Nursing process step: Assessment

Client needs category: Safe, effective care environment

Client needs subcategory: Management of care

Cognitive level: Analysis

---

3. A client returns from the operating room after receiving extensive abdominal surgery. He has 1,000 ml of lactated Ringer's solution infusing via a central line. The physician orders the I.V. fluid to be infused at 125 ml/hour plus the total output of the previous hour. The drip factor of the tubing is 15 gtt/minute and the output for the previous hour was 75 ml via Foley catheter, 50 ml via nasogastric tube, and 10 ml via Jackson Pratt tube. For how many drops per minute should the nurse set the I.V. flow rate to deliver the correct amount of fluid?

_____

ANSWER: 65

Rationale: First, calculate the volume to be infused (in milliliters):

$$75 \text{ ml} + 50 \text{ ml} + 10 \text{ ml} =$$
$$135 \text{ ml total output for the previous hour;}$$

$$135 \text{ ml} + 125 \text{ ml ordered as a constant flow} =$$
$$260 \text{ ml to be infused over the next hour}$$

Next, use the formula:

$$\text{Volume to be infused/Total minutes}$$
$$\text{to be infused} \times \text{Drip factor} = \text{Drops per minute.}$$

In this case,

$$260 \text{ ml} \div 60 \text{ minutes} \times 15 \text{ gtt/minute} =$$
$$65 \text{ gtt/minute}$$

Nursing process step: Implementation

Client needs category: Physiological integrity

Client needs subcategory: Pharmacological and parenteral therapies

Cognitive level: Analysis

4. A client with a retroperitoneal abscess is receiving gentamicin (Garamycin). Which of the following should the nurse monitor?

Select all that apply:

☐ **A.** Hearing

☐ **B.** Urine output

☐ **C.** Hematocrit (HCT)

☐ **D.** Blood urea nitrogen (BUN) and creatinine levels

☐ **E.** Serum calcium level

ANSWER: A, B, D

Rationale: Adverse reactions to gentamicin include ototoxicity and nephrotoxicity. The nurse must monitor the client's hearing and instruct him to report any hearing loss or tinnitus. Signs of nephrotoxicity include decreased urine output and elevated BUN and creatinine levels. Gentamicin doesn't affect the serum calcium level or HCT.

Nursing process step: Assessment

Client needs category: Physiological integrity

Client needs subcategory: Pharmacological and parenteral therapies

Cognitive level: Analysis

---

5. The nurse is assessing the abdomen of a client who was admitted to the emergency department with suspected appendicitis. Identify the area of the abdomen that the nurse should palpate last.

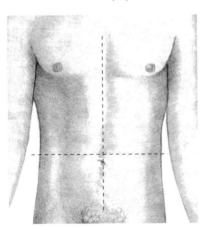

ANSWER:

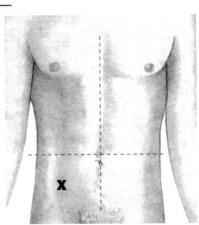

Rationale: An acute attack of appendicitis localizes as pain and tenderness in the lower right quadrant, midway between the umbilicus and the crest of the ilium. This area should be palpated last in order to determine if pain is also present in other areas of the abdomen.

Nursing process step: Assessment

Client needs category: Health promotion and maintenance

Client needs subcategory: Prevention and early detection of disease

Cognitive level: Application

---

6. While preparing a client for an upper GI endoscopy (esophagogastroduodenoscopy), the nurse should implement which of the following interventions?

Select all that apply:

☐ **A.** Administer a preparation to cleanse the GI tract, such as Golytely or Fleets Phospha-Soda.

☐ **B.** Tell the client he shouldn't eat or drink for 6 to 12 hours before the procedure.

☐ **C.** Tell the client he must be on a clear liquid diet for 24 hours before the procedure.

☐ **D.** Inform the client that he'll receive a sedative before the procedure.

☐ **E.** Tell the client that he may eat and drink immediately after the procedure.

ANSWER: B, D

Rationale: The client shouldn't eat or drink for 6 to 12 hours before the procedure to assure that his upper GI tract is clear for viewing. The client will receive a sedative before the endoscope is inserted that will help him relax, but allow him to remain conscious. GI tract cleansing and a clear liquid diet are interventions for a client having a lower GI tract procedure, such as a colonoscopy. Food and fluids must be withheld until the gag reflex returns.

Nursing process step: Implementation

Client needs category: Physiological integrity

Client needs subcategory: Reduction of risk potential

Cognitive level: Application

---

7. The nurse is caring for a client who has had extensive abdominal surgery and is in critical condition. The nurse notes that the complete blood count shows an 8 g/dl hemoglobin and a 30% hematocrit. Dextrose 5% in half-normal saline solution is infusing through a triple lumen central catheter at 125 ml/hour. The physician orders include:

Gentamicin (Garamycin) 80 mg I.V. piggyback in 50 ml D_5W over 30 minutes.
Ranitidine (Zantac) 50 mg I.V. in 50 ml D_5W piggyback over 30 minutes.
One unit of 250 ml of packed RBCs over 3 hours.
Flush the nasogastric tube with 30 ml normal saline every 2 hours.

How many milliliters should the nurse document as the intake for the 8-hour shift?

ANSWER: 1,470

Rationale:

Regular I.V. at 125 ml x 8 hours = 1,000 ml
Gentamicin (Garamycin) piggyback = 50 ml
Ranitidine (Zantac) piggyback = 50 ml
Packed red blood cells = 250 ml
Nasogastric flushes 30 ml x 4 = 120 ml
Total = 1,470 ml

Nursing process step: Implementation

Client needs category: Physiological integrity

Client needs subcategory: Basic care and comfort

Cognitive level: Analysis

8. Indicate the location of an ostomy for which the client could eventually not need to wear an ostomy bag?

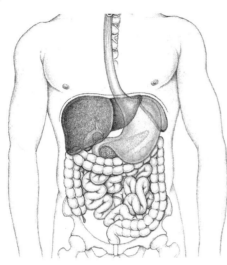

ANSWER:

ANSWER:

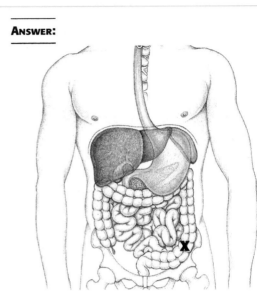

Rationale: With a sigmoid colostomy, the feces are solid; therefore, the client may eventually gain enough control that he would not need to wear a colostomy bag. With a descending colostomy, the feces are semi-mushy. With a transverse colostomy, the feces are mushy. With an ascending colostomy, the feces are fluid. In these three latter cases, it is unlikely that the client could gain control of elimination; consequently, wearing an ostomy bag would be necessary.

Nursing process step: Planning

Client needs category: Physiologic integrity

Client needs subcategory: Basic care and comfort

Cognitive level: Application

---

9. Which of the following findings is common in neonates born with esophageal atresia?

Select all that apply:

☐ **A.** Decreased production of saliva

☐ **B.** Cyanosis

☐ **C.** Coughing

☐ **D.** Inadequate swallow

☐ **E.** Choking

☐ **F.** Inability to cough

ANSWER: B, C, E

Rationale: Cyanosis, coughing, and choking occur when fluid from the blind pouch is aspirated into the trachea. Saliva production doesn't decrease in neonates born with esophageal atresia. The ability to swallow isn't affected by this disorder.

Nursing process step: Assessment

Client needs category: Physiological integrity

Client needs subcategory: Physiological adaptation

Cognitive level: Analysis

---

10. A 28-year-old client is admitted with inflammatory bowel syndrome (Crohn's disease). Which of the following should the nurse expect to be part of the care plan?

Select all that apply:

☐ **A.** Lactulose therapy

☐ **B.** High-fiber diet

☐ **C.** High protein milkshakes

☐ **D.** Corticosteroid therapy

☐ **E.** Antidiarrheal medications

ANSWER: D, E

Rationale: Corticosteroids, such as prednisone, reduce the signs and symptoms of diarrhea, pain, and bleeding by decreasing inflammation. Antidiarrheals, such as diphenoxylate (Lomotil), combat diarrhea by decreasing peristalsis. Lactulose is used to treat chronic constipation and would aggravate the symptoms. A high-fiber diet and milk and milk products are contraindicated in clients with Crohn's disease because they may promote diarrhea.

Nursing process step: Planning

Client needs category: Safe, effective care environment

Client needs subcategory: Management of care

Cognitive level: Analysis

Integumentary disorders

1. A 10-year-old client is brought to the office with complaints of severe itching in both hands that is especially annoying at night. On inspection, the nurse notes gray-brown burrows with epidermal curved ridges and follicular papules. The physician performs a lesion scraping to assess this condition. Based on the signs and symptoms, what diagnosis should the nurse expect?

ANSWER: Scabies

Rationale: The signs and symptoms for scabies include gray-brown burrows, epidermal curved or linear ridges, and follicular papules. Clients complain of severe itching that usually occurs at night. Scabies commonly occurs in school-age children. The most common areas for infestation are the finger webs, flexor surface of the wrists, and antecubital fossae.

Nursing process step: Analysis

Client needs category: Physiological integrity

Client needs subcategory: Physiological adaptation

Cognitive level: Analysis

2. While assessing the skin of a 45-year-old, fair-skinned, female client, the nurse notes a lesion on the medial aspect of her lower leg. It has irregular borders, with various shades of black and brown. The client states that the lesion itches occasionally and bled slightly a few weeks ago. She also reveals a history of sunburns. What kind of lesion do these signs and symptoms point to?

_____

ANSWER: Melanoma

Rationale: The ABCD's of melanoma are Asymmetry of the lesion, Borders that are irregular, Colors that vary in shades, and increased Diameter. Fair skin with a history of sunburn and the location of the lesion on the leg (the most common site in women) are risk factors for melanoma.

Nursing process step: Assessment

Client needs category: Health promotion and maintenance

Client needs subcategory: Prevention and early detection of disease

Cognitive level: Analysis

---

3. While assessing a client with a stage 2 pressure ulcer, the nurse observes which of the following criteria?

Select all that apply:

☐ **A.** The skin is intact.

☐ **B.** There is full-thickness skin loss.

☐ **C.** Undermining is present.

☐ **D.** Sinus tracts have developed.

☐ **E.** The ulcer is superficial like a blister.

☐ **F.** There is partial-thickness skin loss of the epidermis.

ANSWER: E, F

Rationale: A stage 2 pressure ulcer involves partial-thickness skin loss of the epidermis or dermis. The ulcer is superficial and presents clinically as an abrasion, blister, or shallow crater. Intact skin is a characteristic of a stage 1 pressure ulcer. Full-thickness skin loss, undermining, and sinus tracts are characteristics of a stage 3 pressure ulcer.

Nursing process step: Assessment

Client needs category: Physiological integrity

Client needs subcategory: Physiological adaptation

Cognitive level: Analysis

4. The nurse is planning the care for a client with a pressure ulcer. Which of the following statements should the nurse include in the client's nursing care plan?

Select all that apply:

☐ **A.** Use pressure reduction devices.

☐ **B.** Increase carbohydrates in the diet.

☐ **C.** Reposition every 1 to 2 hours.

☐ **D.** Teach the family how to care for the wound.

☐ **E.** Clean the area around the ulcer with mild soap.

☐ **F.** Avoid the use of support-surface therapy.

ANSWER: A, C, D, E

Rationale: Using a pressure reduction device, repositioning every 2 hours, and cleaning the area around the wound with a mild soap will aid in healing or will prevent further skin breakdown. Teaching the family how to care for the wound will assist with discharge planning. Protein, not carbohydrate, intake, should be increased to promote wound healing. Support-surface therapy is a major therapeutic method of managing pressure, friction, and shear on tissues.

Nursing process step: Planning

Client needs category: Physiological integrity

Client needs subcategory: Basic care and comfort

Cognitive level: Analysis

---

5. The triage nurse in the emergency room admits a 50-year-old male client with second-degree burns on the anterior and posterior portions of both legs. Based on the rule of nines, what percentage of the body is burned?

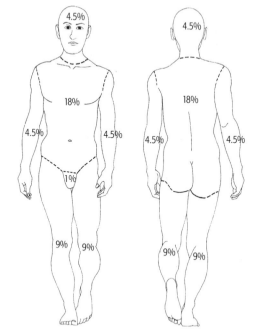

ANSWER: 36

Rationale: The anterior and posterior portion of one leg is 18%. If both legs are burned, the total is 36%.

Nursing process step: Assessment

Client needs category: Physiological integrity

Client needs subcategory: Physiological adaptation

Cognitive level: Analysis

6. A client returns from the operating room with a partial-thickness skin graft on her left arm. The donor tissue was taken from her left hip. In planning her immediate postoperative care, which of the following interventions should the nurse include?

Select all that apply:

☐ **A.** Change the dressing every 8 hours on the graft site.

☐ **B.** Elevate the left arm and provide complete rest of the grafted area.

☐ **C.** Administer pain medication every 4 hours as ordered for pain in donor site.

☐ **D.** Perform range-of-motion (ROM) exercises to the left arm every 4 hours.

☐ **E.** Monitor the pulse in the left arm every 4 hours.

☐ **F.** Encourage the client to ambulate as desired the first postoperative day.

ANSWER: B, C, E

Rationale: The left arm should be elevated to reduce edema. Complete rest of the arm is needed to allow the graft to adhere. The donor site is usually more painful than the graft site and the client will require pain medication to obtain relief. Because adequate circulation is needed for graft healing, it's important to monitor for pulse presence. Changing the dressing every 8 hours, performing ROM exercises, and ambulating are inappropriate because postoperative graft sites require immobilization for 3 to 5 days.

Nursing process step: Planning

Client needs category: Physiological integrity

Client needs subcategory: Physiological adaptation

Cognitive level: Application

Immune and hematologic disorders

1. A client with systemic lupus erythematosus has the classic rash of lesions on the cheeks and bridge of the nose. What term does the nurse use to describe this characteristic pattern in her documentation?

ANSWER: Butterfly

Rationale: In the classic lupus rash, lesions appear on the cheeks and the bridge of the nose, creating a characteristic butterfly pattern. The rash may vary in severity from malar erythema to discoid lesions (plaque).

Nursing process step: Assessment

Client needs category: Physiological integrity

Client needs subcategory: Physiological adaptation

Cognitive level: Comprehension

2. A client must receive a blood transfusion of packed red blood cells for severe anemia. What I.V. fluid should the nurse use to prime the tubing before hanging this blood product?

_____

ANSWER: Normal saline solution

Rationale: Normal saline solution is used for administering blood transfusions. Lactated Ringer's solution or dextrose solutions may cause blood clotting or red blood cell hemolysis.

Nursing process step: Implementation

Client needs category: Physiological integrity

Client needs subcategory: Pharmacological and parenteral therapies

Cognitive level: Application

---

3. The nurse is planning care for a client with human immunodeficiency virus (HIV). She's being assisted by a licensed practical nurse (LPN). Which statements by the LPN indicate her understanding of HIV transmission?

Select all that apply:

☐ **A.** "I'll wear a gown, mask, and gloves for all client contact."

☐ **B.** "I don't need to wear any personal protective equipment because nurses have a low risk of occupational exposure."

☐ **C.** "I'll wear a mask if the client has a cough caused by an upper respiratory infection."

☐ **D.** "I'll wear a mask, gown, and gloves when splashing of body fluids is likely."

☐ **E.** "I will wash my hands after client care."

ANSWER: D, E

Rationale: Standard precautions include wearing gloves for any known or anticipated contact with blood, body fluids, tissue, mucous membranes, or nonintact skin. If the task may result in splashing or splattering of blood or body fluids to the face, a mask and goggles or face shield should be worn. If the task may result in splashing or splattering of blood or body fluids to the body, a fluid-resistant gown or apron should be worn. Hands should be washed before and after client care and after removing gloves. A gown, mask, and gloves aren't necessary for client care unless contact with body fluids, tissue, mucous membranes, or nonintact skin is expected. Nurses have an increased, not decreased, risk of occupational exposure to blood-borne pathogens. HIV isn't transmitted in sputum unless blood is present.

Nursing process step: Planning

Client needs category: Safe, effective care environment

Client needs subcategory: Safety and infection control

Cognitive level: Application

4. Which nonpharmacologic interventions should the nurse include in the care plan for a client who has moderate rheumatoid arthritis?

Select all that apply:

☐ **A.** Massaging inflamed joints

☐ **B.** Avoiding range-of-motion exercises

☐ **C.** Applying splints to inflamed joints

☐ **D.** Using assistive devices at all times

☐ **E.** Selecting clothing that has Velcro fasteners

☐ **F.** Applying moist heat to joints

ANSWER: C, E, F

Rationale: Supportive, nonpharmacologic measures for the client with rheumatoid arthritis include applying splints to rest inflamed joints, using Velcro fasteners on clothes to aid in dressing, and applying moist heat to joints to relax muscles and relieve pain. Inflamed joints should never be massaged because doing so can aggravate inflammation. A physical therapy program including range-of-motion exercises and carefully individualized therapeutic exercises prevents loss of joint function. Assistive devices should only be used when marked loss of range of motion occurs.

Nursing process step: Planning

Client needs category: Physiological integrity

Client needs subcategory: Basic care and comfort

Cognitive level: Application

---

5. The nurse is assessing a client with a suspected Epstein-Barr viral infection. Identify the quadrant of the abdomen where the nurse is best able to palpate the spleen.

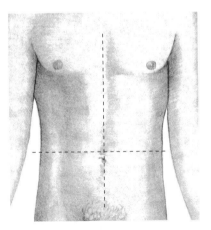

ANSWER:

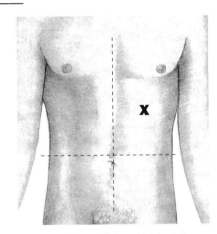

Rationale: The spleen is located in the left upper quadrant of the abdomen. It's posterior and slightly inferior to the stomach. The nurse should stop palpating immediately if she feels the spleen because compression can cause rupture.

Nursing process step: Assessment

Client needs category: Physiological integrity

Client needs subcategory: Physiological adaptation

Cognitive level: Application

6. A client has a viral infection and swollen lymph nodes. Identify the area where the nurse should place her hand to palpate the submandibular lymph nodes?

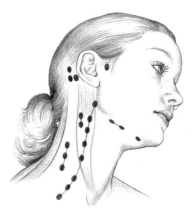

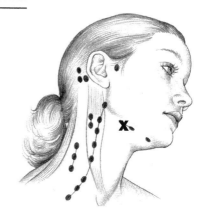

Rationale: The submandibular lymph nodes are found halfway between the angle and tip of the mandible.

Nursing process step: Assessment

Client needs category: Physiological integrity

Client needs subcategory: Physiological adaptation

Cognitive level: Application

Endocrine and metabolic disorders

1. A 56-year-old female client is being discharged after having a thyroidectomy. Which of the following discharge instructions would be appropriate for this client?

Select all that apply:

☐ **A.** Report signs and symptoms of hypoglycemia.

☐ **B.** Take thyroid replacement medication as ordered.

☐ **C.** Watch for changes in body functioning, such as lethargy, restlessness, sensitivity to cold, and dry skin, and report these changes to the physician.

☐ **D.** Recognize the signs of dehydration.

☐ **E.** Avoid all over-the-counter medications.

☐ **F.** Carry injectable dexamethasone at all times.

ANSWER: B, C

Rationale: After the removal of the thyroid gland, the client needs to take thyroid replacement medication. The client also needs to report such changes as lethargy, restlessness, cold sensitivity, and dry skin, which may indicate the need for a higher dosage of medication. The thyroid gland doesn't regulate blood glucose level; therefore, signs and symptoms of hypoglycemia aren't relevant for this client. Dehydration is seen in diabetes insipidus. Injectable dexamethasone isn't needed for this client.

Nursing process step: Implementation

Client needs category: Physiological integrity

Client needs subcategory: Physiological adaptation

Cognitive level: Application

2. A client is admitted with a diagnosis of diabetic ketoacidosis. An insulin drip is initiated with 50 U of insulin in 100 ml of normal saline solution. The I.V. is being infused via an infusion pump and the pump is currently set at 10 ml/hour. The nurse determines that the client is receiving how many units of insulin each hour?

_____

ANSWER: 5

Rationale: To determine the number of insulin units the client is receiving per hour, the nurse must first determine the number of units in each ml of fluid (50 U ÷ 100 ml = 0.5 U/ml). Next, she multiplies the units/ml by the rate of ml/hour (0.5 units × 10 ml/hr = 5 U).

Nursing process step: Analysis

Client needs category: Physiological integrity

Client needs subcategory: Pharmacological and parenteral therapies

Cognitive level: Application

3. A client in the emergency department reports that he has been vomiting excessively for the past 2 days. His arterial blood gas analysis shows a pH of 7.50, $Paco_2$ of 43 mm Hg, Pao_2 of 75 mm Hg, and HCO_3^- of 42 mEq/L. Based on these findings, the nurse documents that the patient is experiencing which acid-base imbalance?

_____

ANSWER: Metabolic alkalosis

Rationale: A pH over 7.45 with a bicarbonate level over 26 mEq/L indicates metabolic alkalosis. Metabolic alkalosis is always secondary to an underlying cause and is marked by decreased amounts of acid or increased amounts of base bicarbonate.

Nursing process step: Implementation

Client needs category: Physiological integrity

Client needs subcategory: Physiological adaptation

Cognitive level: Analysis

4. The nurse is performing an admission assessment on a client who has been diagnosed with diabetes insipidus. Which of the following findings should the nurse expect to note during the assessment?

Select all that apply:

☐ **A.** Extreme polyuria

☐ **B.** Excessive thirst

☐ **C.** Elevated systolic blood pressure

☐ **D.** Low urine specific gravity

☐ **E.** Bradycardia

☐ **F.** Elevated serum potassium level

ANSWER: A, B, D

Rationale: Signs and symptoms of diabetes insipidus include an abrupt onset of extreme polyuria, excessive thirst, dry skin and mucous membranes, tachycardia, and hypotension. Diagnostic studies reveal low urine specific gravity and osmolarity and elevated serum sodium. Serum potassium levels are likely to be decreased, not increased.

Nursing process step: Assessment

Client needs category: Physiological integrity

Client needs subcategory: Physiological adaptation

Cognitive level: Comprehension

---

5. A client is being treated for hypothyroidism. The nurse knows that thyroid replacement therapy has been inadequate when she notes which of the following findings?

Select all that apply:

☐ **A.** Prolonged QT interval on electrocardiogram

☐ **B.** Tachycardia

☐ **C.** Low body temperature

☐ **D.** Nervousness

☐ **E.** Bradycardia

☐ **F.** Dry mouth

ANSWER: A, C, E

Rationale: In hypothyroidism, the body is in a hypometabolic state. Therefore, a prolonged QT interval with bradycardia and subnormal body temperature would indicate that replacement therapy was inadequate. Tachycardia, nervousness, and dry mouth are symptoms of an excessive level of thyroid hormone; these findings would indicate that the client has received an excessive dose of thyroid hormone.

Nursing process step: Analysis

Client needs category: Physiological integrity

Client needs subcategory: Reduction of risk potential

Cognitive level: Analysis

6. A 55-year-old diabetic client is admitted with hypoglycemia. Which information should the nurse include in her client teaching?

Select all that apply:

☐ **A.** Hypoglycemia can result from excessive alcohol consumption.

☐ **B.** Skipping meals can cause hypoglycemia.

☐ **C.** Symptoms of hypoglycemia include thirst and excessive urinary output.

☐ **D.** Strenuous activity may result in hypoglycemia.

☐ **E.** Symptoms of hypoglycemia include shakiness, confusion, and headache.

☐ **F.** Hypoglycemia is a relatively harmless situation.

ANSWER: A, B, D, E

Rationale: Alcohol consumption, missed meals, and strenuous activity may lead to hypoglycemia. Symptoms of hypoglycemia include shakiness, confusion, headache, sweating, and tingling sensations around the mouth. Thirst and excessive urination are symptoms of hyperglycemia. Hypoglycemia can become a life-threatening disorder involving seizures and death to brain cells; the client shouldn't be told that the condition is relatively harmless.

Nursing process step: Implementation

Client needs category: Physiological integrity

Client needs subcategory: Reduction of risk potential

Cognitive level: Application

---

7. A 20-year-old client comes to the clinic because she has experienced a weight loss of 20 lb over the last month, even though her appetite has been "ravenous" and she hasn't changed her activity level. She's diagnosed with Grave's disease. Which other signs and symptoms support the diagnosis of Grave's disease?

Select all that apply:

☐ **A.** Rapid, bounding pulse

☐ **B.** Bradycardia

☐ **C.** Heat intolerance

☐ **D.** Mild tremors

☐ **E.** Nervousness

☐ **F.** Constipation

ANSWER: A, C, D, E

Rationale: Grave's disease, or hyperthyroidism, is a hypermetabolic state that's associated with rapid, bounding pulses; heat intolerance; tremors; and nervousness. Bradycardia and constipation are signs and symptoms of hypothyroidism.

Nursing process step: Analysis

Client needs category: Health promotion and maintenance

Client needs subcategory: Prevention and early detection of disease

Cognitive level: Analysis

8. A client with Addison's disease is scheduled for discharge after being hospitalized for an adrenal crisis. Which statements by the client would indicate that client teaching has been effective?

Select all that apply:

☐ **A.** "I have to take my steroids for 10 days."

☐ **B.** "I need to weigh myself daily to be sure I don't eat too many calories."

☐ **C.** "I need to call my doctor to discuss my steroid needs before I have dental work."

☐ **D.** "I will call the doctor if I suddenly feel profoundly weak or dizzy."

☐ **E.** "If I feel like I have the flu, I'll carry on as usual because this is an expected response."

☐ **F.** "I need to obtain and wear a Medic Alert Bracelet."

ANSWER: C, D, F

Rationale: Dental work can be a cause of physical stress; therefore, the client's physician needs to be informed about the dental work and an adjusted dosage of steroids may be necessary. Fatigue, weakness, and dizziness are symptoms of inadequate dosing of steroid therapy; the physician should be notified if these symptoms occur. A Medic Alert bracelet allows health care providers to access the client's history of Addison's disease if the client is unable to communicate this information. A client with Addison's disease doesn't produce enough steroids, so routine administration of steroids is a lifetime treatment. Daily weights should be monitored to monitor changes in fluid balance, not calorie intake. Influenza is an added physical stressor and the client may require an increased dosage of steroids. The client shouldn't "carry on as usual."

Nursing process step: Evaluation

Client needs category: Physiological integrity

Client needs subcategory: Reduction of risk potential

Cognitive level: Analysis

---

9. A businesswoman comes into the clinic with a progressively enlarging neck. The client mentions that she has been in a foreign country for the last 3 months and that she didn't eat much while she was there because she didn't like the food. The client also mentions that she becomes dizzy when lifting her arms to do normal household chores or dressing. What endocrine disorder would you expect the physician to diagnose?

ANSWER: Goiter

Rationale: A goiter can result from inadequate dietary intake of iodine associated with changes in foods or malnutrition. It's caused by insufficient thyroid gland production and depletion of glandular iodine. Signs and symptoms of this malfunction include enlargement of the thyroid gland, dizziness when raising the arms above the head, dysphagia, and respiratory distress.

Nursing process step: Assessment

Client needs category: Physiological integrity

Client needs subcategory: Physiological adaptation

Cognitive level: Comprehension

10. A client who suffered a brain injury after falling off a ladder has recently developed syndrome of inappropriate antidiuretic hormone (SIADH). What findings indicate that the treatment he's receiving for SIADH is effective?

Select all that apply:

☐ **A.** Decrease in body weight

☐ **B.** Rise in blood pressure and drop in heart rate

☐ **C.** Absence of wheezes in the lungs

☐ **D.** Increase in urine output

☐ **E.** Decrease in urine osmolarity

ANSWER: A, D, E

Rationale: SIADH is an abnormality involving an excessive release of antidiuretic hormone. The predominant feature is water retention with oliguria, edema and weight gain. Successful treatment should result in a reduction in weight, increased urine output, and a decrease in the urine concentration (urine osmolarity).

Nursing process step: Evaluation

Client needs category: Physiologic integrity

Client needs subcategory: Physiological adaptation

Cognitive level: Analysis

---

11. A nurse is about to administer a client's morning dosage of insulin. The client's order is for 5 U of regular and 10 U of NPH given as a basal dose. He also is to receive an amount prescribed from his medium dose sliding scale (shown below) based on his morning blood glucose level. The nurse performs a bedside blood glucose measurement and the result is 264 mg/dl. How many total units of insulin should the nurse administer to the client?

Plasma glucose (mg/dl)	Low dose (Regular insulin)	Medium dose (Regular insulin)	High dose (Regular insulin)	Very high dose (Regular insulin)
< 70	← Call physician →			
71-140	0 U	0 U	0 U	0 U
141-180	1 U	2 U	4 U	10 U
181-240	2 U	4 U	8 U	15 U
241-300	4 U	6 U	12 U	20 U
301-400	6 U	9 U	16 U	25 U
> 400	8 U	12 U	20 U	30 U
	← and call physician →			

ANSWER: 21

Rationale: The basal dosage for this client is 5 U of regular insulin and 10 U of NPH insulin. Using the medium dose sliding scale and the client's blood glucose reading of 264 mg/dl, the nurse should determine that an additional 6 U of regular insulin are required, totalling 21 U (5 U + 10 U + 6 U = 21 U).

Nursing process step: Implementation

Client needs category: Physiological integrity

Client needs subcategory: Pharmacological and parenteral therapies

Cognitive level: Application

12. A client is seen in the clinic with a possible parathormone deficiency. Diagnosis of this condition includes the analysis of serum electrolytes. Which of the following electrolytes would the nurse expect to be abnormal?

Select all that apply:

☐ **A.** Sodium

☐ **B.** Potassium

☐ **C.** Calcium

☐ **D.** Chloride

☐ **E.** Glucose

☐ **F.** Phosphorous

ANSWER: C, F

Rationale: A client with a parathormone deficiency has abnormal calcium and phosphorous values because parathormone regulates these two electrolytes. Potassium, chloride, sodium, and glucose aren't affected by a parathormone deficiency.

Nursing process step: Evaluation

Client needs category: Health promotion and maintenance

Client needs subcategory: Prevention and early detection of disease

Cognitive level: Analysis

Musculoskeletal disorders

1. A client is diagnosed with osteoporosis. Which statements should the nurse include when teaching the client about the disease?

Select all that apply:

☐ **A.** It's common in females after menopause.

☐ **B.** It's a degenerative disease characterized by a decrease in bone density.

☐ **C.** It's a congenital disease caused by poor dietary intake of milk products.

☐ **D.** It can cause pain and injury.

☐ **E.** Passive range-of-motion exercises can promote bone growth.

☐ **F.** Weight-bearing exercise should be avoided.

ANSWER: A, B, D

Rationale: Osteoporosis is a degenerative metabolic bone disorder in which the rate of bone resorption accelerates and the rate of bone formation decelerates, thus decreasing bone density. Postmenopausal women are at increased risk for this disorder because of the loss of estrogen. The decrease in bone density can cause pain and injury. Osteoporosis isn't a congenital disorder; however, low calcium intake does contribute to the disorder. Passive range-of-motion exercises may be performed but they won't promote bone growth. The client should be encouraged to participate in weight-bearing exercise because it promotes bone growth.

Nursing process step: Implementation

Client needs category: Physiological integrity

Client needs subcategory: Physiological adaptation

Cognitive level: Application

2. A 72-year-old female client reports that she has lost an inch in height over the past 15 years. The nurse explains to the client that she has a musculoskeletal disorder. What's this disorder called?

_____

Rationale: Osteoporosis, a degenerative disease characterized by a decrease in bone density, typically occurs in postmenopausal woman. A client with osteoporosis may report a gradual loss in height after menopause.

Nursing process step: Implementation

Client needs category: Health promotion and maintenance

Client needs subcategory: Prevention and early detection of disease

Cognitive level: Comprehension

3. A client is diagnosed with gout. Which foods should the nurse instruct the client to avoid?

Select all that apply:

☐ **A.** Green leafy vegetables

☐ **B.** Liver

☐ **C.** Cod

☐ **D.** Chocolate

☐ **E.** Sardines

☐ **F.** Eggs

ANSWER: B, C, E

Rationale: Clients with gout should avoid foods that are high in purines, such as liver, cod, and sardines. They should also avoid anchovies, kidneys, sweetbreads, lentils, and alcoholic beverages — especially beer and wine. Green leafy vegetables, chocolate, and eggs aren't high in purines.

Nursing process step: Implementation

Client needs category: Physiological integrity

Client needs subcategory: Basic care and comfort

Cognitive level: Application

4 An elderly client fell and fractured the neck of his femur. Identify the area where the fracture occurred.

ANSWER:

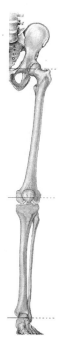

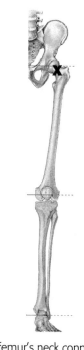

Rationale: The femur's neck connects the femur's round ball head to the shaft.

Nursing process step: Assessment

Client needs category: Physiological integrity

Client needs subcategory: Physiological adaptation

Cognitive level: Comprehension

---

5. A client is in the emergency department with a suspected fracture of the right hip. Which assessment findings of the right leg would the nurse expect?

Select all that apply:

☐ **A.** The right leg is longer than the left leg.

☐ **B.** The right leg is shorter than the left leg.

☐ **C.** The right leg is abducted.

☐ **D.** The right leg is adducted.

☐ **E.** The right leg is externally rotated.

☐ **F.** The right leg is internally rotated.

ANSWER: B, D, E

Rationale: In a hip fracture, the affected leg is shorter, adducted, and externally rotated.

Nursing process step: Assessment

Client needs category: Physiological integrity

Client needs subcategory: Physiological adaptation

Cognitive level: Application

6. A client is scheduled for a laminectomy of the L1 and L2 vertebrae. Identify the area that's involved in the client's surgery.

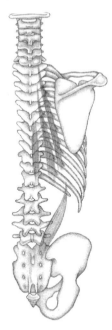

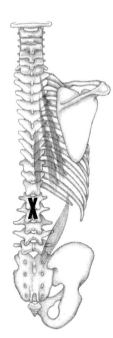

Rationale: In laminectomy, one or more of the bony laminae that cover the vertebrae are removed. There are five lumbar vertebrae and they are numbered from top to bottom. L5 is the closest to the sacrum. Count up from the sacrum to locate L1 and L2.

Nursing process step: Implementation

Client needs category: Physiological integrity

Client needs subcategory: Physiologic adaptation

Cognitive level: Comprehension

---

7. The nurse is assisting a client with range-of-motion exercises. The nurse moves the client's leg out and away from the midline of the body. What movement does the nurse document?

ANSWER: Abduction

Rationale: Movement away from the body or midline is called abduction. Movement toward the midline is called adduction.

Nursing process step: Implementation

Client needs category: Physiological integrity

Client needs subcategory: Basic care and comfort

Cognitive level: Comprehension

1. The nurse is preparing a female client with tonic-clonic seizure disorder for discharge. Which instructions should the nurse include about phenytoin (Dilantin)?

Select all that apply:

☐ **A.** Monitor for skin rash.

☐ **B.** Maintain adequate amounts of fluid and fiber in the diet.

☐ **C.** Perform good oral hygiene, including daily brushing and flossing.

☐ **D.** Receive necessary periodic blood work.

☐ **E.** Report to the physician any problems with walking, coordination, slurred speech, or nausea.

☐ **F.** Feel safe about taking this drug, even during pregnancy.

ANSWER: A, C, D, E

Rationale: A rash may occur 10 to 14 days after starting phenytoin. If a rash appears, the client should notify the physician and discontinue the medication. Because phenytoin may cause gingival hyperplasia, the client must practice good oral hygiene and see a dentist regularly. Periodic blood work is necessary to monitor complete blood counts, platelet levels, hepatic function, and drug levels. Signs and symptoms of phenytoin toxicity include problems with walking, coordination, slurred speech, and nausea. Other signs of toxicity include lethargy, diplopia, nystagmus, and disturbances in balance. These symptoms must be reported to the physician immediately. While adequate amounts of fluid and fiber are part of a healthy diet, they aren't required for a client taking phenytoin. Phenytoin must be used cautiously during pregnancy because of the increased incidence of birth defects; phenobarbital is a safer drug to take during pregnancy.

Nursing process step: Implementation

Client needs category: Physiological integrity

Client needs subcategory: Pharmacological and parenteral therapies

Cognitive level: Application

2. A client is undergoing testing to confirm a diagnosis of myasthenia gravis. The nurse explains that myasthenia gravis is established if muscle function improves after the client receives an I.V. injection of a medication. What is the brand-name medication the nurse tells the client he'll receive during this test?

ANSWER: Tensilon

Rationale: The most useful and reliable diagnostic test in the diagnosis of myasthenia gravis is the Tensilon test. Within 30 to 60 seconds following injection of Tensilon, most clients with myasthenia gravis will demonstrate a marked improvement in muscle tone that lasts about 4 to 5 minutes.

Nursing process step: Implementation

Client needs category: Physiological integrity

Client needs subcategory: Pharmacological and parenteral therapies

Cognitive level: Application

3. The nurse is assessing a client with meningitis. The nurse places the client in a supine position and flexes the client's leg at the hip and knee. The nurse notes resistance when straightening the knee and the client reports pain. The nurse documents what neurologic sign as positive?

_____

ANSWER: Kernig's

_____

Rationale: A positive Kernig's sign is a manifestation of meningeal irritation. The nurse can elicit this sign by placing the client in a supine position and flexing the leg at the hip and knee. Pain or resistance when the knee is straightened suggests meningeal irritation.

Nursing process step: Assessment

Client needs category: Physiological integrity

Client needs subcategory: Physiological adaptation

Cognitive level: Application

---

4. The nurse is assessing a client's extraocular eye movements as part of the neurologic examination. Which of the following cranial nerves is the nurse assessing?

Select all that apply:

☐ **A.** Cranial nerve II

☐ **B.** Cranial nerve III

☐ **C.** Cranial nerve IV

☐ **D.** Cranial nerve V

☐ **E.** Cranial nerve VI

☐ **F.** Cranial nerve VIII

ANSWER: B, C, E

_____

Rationale: Assessing extraocular eye movements helps evaluate the function of cranial nerves III (oculomotor), IV (trochlear), and VI (abducens). The oculomotor nerve originates in the brainstem and controls the movement of the eyeball up, down, and inward; raises the eyelid; and constricts the pupil. The trochlear nerve rotates the eyeball downward and outward. The abducens nerve originates in the pons and rotates the eyeball laterally. Assessing the client's vision helps evaluation of cranial nerve II. Cranial nerve V, the trigeminal nerve, has three branches: assessing sensation of the cornea (corneal reflex) helps the nurse evaluate the ophthalmic branch functions; assessing sensation to the skin of the cheek, upper jaw, teeth, lips, hard palate, maxillary sinus, and part of the nasal mucosa helps the nurse evaluate the maxillary branch functions; and assessing sensation to the skin of the lower lip, chin, ear, mucous membrane, teeth of the lower jaw, and tongue helps the nurse evaluate the mandibular branch functions. Assessing hearing (cochlear) and balance (vestibular) helps evaluation of cranial nerve VIII, the acoustic nerve.

Nursing process step: Assessment

Client needs category: Physiological integrity

Client needs subcategory: Physiological adaptation

Cognitive level: Analysis

5. The nurse is assessing the level of consciousness of a client who suffered a head injury. She uses the Glasgow Coma Scale and determines that the client's score is 15. Which of the following responses did the nurse assess in this client?

Select all that apply:

☐ **A.** Spontaneous eye opening

☐ **B.** Tachypnea, bradycardia, and hypotension

☐ **C.** Unequal pupil size

☐ **D.** Orientation to person, place, and time

☐ **E.** Motor response to pain localized

☐ **F.** Incomprehensible sounds

ANSWER: A, D

Rationale: The Glasgow Coma Scale assesses level of consciousness by testing and scoring three observations: eye opening, motor response, and verbal stimuli response. Clients are scored on their best responses and these scores are totaled. The highest score is 15. The highest responses in these three categories are spontaneous eye opening; obeying motor commands; and orientation to time, place, and person. Changes in vital signs and unequal pupil size occur with increased intracranial pressure but aren't part of the Glasgow Coma Scale. Incomprehensible verbal response is a score of 2 on the Glasgow Coma Scale, and therefore couldn't contribute to a score of 15.

Nursing process step: Analysis

Client needs category: Physiological integrity

Client needs subcategory: Physiological adaptation

Cognitive level: Analysis

---

6. The nurse is assessing a 2-year-old client diagnosed with bacterial meningitis. Which of the following signs and symptoms of meningeal irritation is the nurse likely to observe?

Select all that apply:

☐ **A.** Generalized seizures

☐ **B.** Nuchal rigidity

☐ **C.** Positive Brudzinski's sign

☐ **D.** Positive Kernig's sign

☐ **E.** Babinski reflex

☐ **F.** Photophobia

ANSWER: B, C, D, F

Rationale: Signs of meningeal irritation include nuchal rigidity, positive Brudzinski's and Kernig's signs, and photophobia. Other signs of meningeal irritation are exaggerated and symmetrical deep tendon reflexes, as well as opisthotonos (a spasm in which the back and extremities arch backward so that the body rests on the head and heals). Generalized seizures, which may accompany meningitis, are caused by irritation to the cerebral cortex, not meningeal irritation. Babinski reflex is a reflex action of the toes that reflects corticospinal tract disease in adults.

Nursing process step: Assessment

Client needs category: Physiological integrity

Client needs subcategory: Physiological adaptation

Cognitive level: Application

7. The nurse is caring for a client with a T5 complete spinal cord injury. Upon assessment, the nurse notes flushed skin, diaphoresis above T5, and a blood pressure of 162/96. The client reports a severe, pounding headache. Which of the following nursing interventions would be appropriate for this client?

Select all that apply:

☐ **A.** Elevate the head of the bed 90 degrees.

☐ **B.** Loosen constrictive clothing.

☐ **C.** Use a fan to reduce diaphoresis.

☐ **D.** Assess for bladder distention and bowel impaction.

☐ **E.** Administer antihypertensive medication.

☐ **F.** Place the client in a supine position with legs elevated.

ANSWER: A, B, D, E

Rationale: The client is exhibiting signs and symptoms of autonomic dysreflexia. The condition is a potentially life-threatening emergency caused by an uninhibited response from the sympathetic nervous system resulting from a lack of control over the autonomic nervous system. The nurse should immediately elevate the head of the bed to 90 degrees and place the extremities in a dependent position to decrease venous return to the heart and increase venous return from the brain. Because tactile stimuli can trigger autonomic dysreflexia, any constrictive clothing should be loosened. The nurse should also assess for distended bladder and bowel impaction — which may trigger autonomic dysreflexia — and correct any problems. Elevated blood pressure is the most life-threatening complication of autonomic dysreflexia because it can cause stroke, myocardial infarction, or seizure activity. If removing the triggering event doesn't reduce the client's blood pressure, I.V. antihypertensives should be administered. A fan shouldn't be used because drafts of cold may trigger autonomic dysreflexia.

Nursing process step: Implementation

Client needs category: Physiological integrity

Client needs subcategory: Reduction of risk potential

Cognitive level: Application

---

8. The nurse is performing a neurologic assessment on a client. The nurse observes the client's tongue for symmetry, tremors, and strength, and assesses the client's speech. What's the number of the cranial nerve that the nurse is assessing?

ANSWER: XII

Rationale: Cranial nerve XII, the hypoglossal nerve, controls tongue movements involved in swallowing and speech. The tongue should be midline, symmetrical, and free of tremors or fasciculations. The nurse tests tongue strength by asking the client to push his tongue against his cheek as the nurse applies resistance. To test the client's speech, the nurse can ask him to repeat the sentence, "Round the rugged rock that ragged rascal ran."

Nursing process step: Assessment

Client needs category: Physiological integrity

Client needs subcategory: Physiological adaptation

Cognitive level: Analysis

9. A 64-year-old client has a cerebral aneurysm. The physician orders hydralazine (Apresoline) 15 mg I.V. every 4 hours as needed to keep the systolic blood pressure less than 140 mm Hg. The label on the hydralazine vial reads *hydralazine 20 mg/ml.* To administer the correct dose, how many milliliters of medication should the nurse draw up in the syringe?

_____

ANSWER: 0.75

Rationale: The following formula is used to calculate drug dosages:

Dose on hand/Quantity on hand = Dose desired/X

Plug in the values for this equation:

20 mg/ml = 15 mg/X = 0.75 ml

Nursing process: Implementation

Client needs category: Physiological integrity

Client needs subcategory: Pharmacological therapies

Cognitive level: Application

---

10. A 45-year-old client is admitted with excruciating paroxysmal facial pain. He reports that the episodes occur most often after feeling cold drafts and drinking cold beverages. Based on these findings, the nurse determines that the client is most likely suffering from which neurologic disorder?

_____

ANSWER: Trigeminal neuralgia

Rationale: Trigeminal neuralgia is a painful disorder of one or more branches of cranial nerve V (trigeminal) that produces paroxysmal attacks of excruciating facial pain. Attacks are precipitated by stimulation of a trigger zone on the face. Triggering events may include light touch to a hypersensitive area, a draft of air, exposure to heat or cold, eating, smiling, talking, or drinking hot or cold beverages. It occurs most commonly in people older than age 40.

Nursing process step: Analysis

Client needs category: Physiological integrity

Client needs subcategory: Physiological adaptation

Cognitive level: Analysis

11. A client is diagnosed with a brain tumor. The nurse's assessment reveals that the client has difficulty interpreting visual stimuli. Based on these findings, the nurse suspects injury to which lobe of the brain?

_____

ANSWER: OCCIPITAL

Rationale: The occipital lobe is responsible for interpreting visual stimuli.

Nursing process step: Assessment

Client needs category: Physiological integrity

Client needs subcategory: Physiological adaptation

Cognitive level: Application

---

12. A client is experiencing problems with balance, as well as fine and gross motor function. Which area of the brain is malfunctioning?

ANSWER:

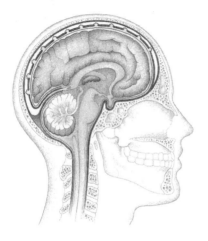

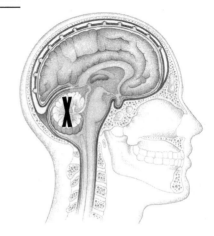

Rationale: The cerebellum is the portion of the brain that controls balance and fine and gross motor function.

Nursing process step: Assessment

Client needs category: Physiological integrity

Client needs subcategory: Reduction of risk potential

Cognitive level: Comprehension

13. The nurse is performing a neurologic assessment on a client during a routine physical examination. To assess the Babinski reflex, indicate the point where the nurse would place the tongue blade to begin the stroke of the foot.

ANSWER:

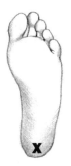

Rationale: To test for the Babinski reflex, use a tongue blade to slowly stroke the lateral side of the under side of the foot. Start at the heel and move towards the great toe. The normal response in an adult is plantar flexion of the toes. Upward movement of the great toe and fanning of the little toes, called the Babinski reflex, is abnormal.

Nursing process step: Assessment

Client needs category: Health promotion and maintenance

Client needs subcategory: Growth and development through the life span

Cognitive level: Comprehension

Respiratory disorders

1. A client who has just had a triple lumen catheter placed in his right subclavian vein complains of chest pain and shortness of breath. His blood pressure is decreased from baseline and, on auscultation of his chest, the nurse notes unequal breath sounds. A chest X-ray is immediately ordered by the physician. What diagnosis should the nurse suspect?

ANSWER: Pneumothorax

Rationale: Pneumothorax (air in the pleural space) is a potential complication of all central venous access devices. Signs and symptoms include chest pain, dyspnea, shoulder or neck pain, irritability, palpitations, light-headedness, hypotension, cyanosis, and unequal breath sounds. A chest X-ray reveals the collapse of the affected lung that results from pneumothorax.

Nursing process step: Analysis

Client needs category: Physiological integrity

Client needs subcategory: Pharmacological and parenteral therapies

Cognitive level: Application

2. A nurse is completing her annual cardiopulmonary resuscitation training. The class instructor tells her that a client has fallen off a ladder and is lying on his back; he is unconscious and is not breathing. What maneuver should the nurse use to open his airway?

_____

ANSWER: Jaw-thrust

Rationale: If a neck or spine injury is suspected, the jaw-thrust maneuver should be used to open the client's airway. To perform this maneuver, the nurse should position herself at the client's head and rest her thumbs on his lower jaw near the corners of the mouth. She should then grasp the angles of his lower jaw with her fingers and lift it forward.

Nursing process step: Analysis

Client needs category: Physiological integrity

Client needs subcategory: Reduction of risk potential

Cognitive level: Analysis

---

3. A nurse is performing a respiratory assessment on a client with pneumonia. She asks the client to say "ninety-nine" several times. Through her stethoscope, she hears the words clearly over his left lower lobe. What term should the nurse use to document this finding?

_____

ANSWER: Bronchophony

Rationale: Bronchophony is an increased intensity and clarity of voice sounds heard over a bronchus surrounded by consolidated lung tissue. Over normal lung tissue, the words are unintelligible; however, over areas of tissue consolidation, such as with pneumonia, the words are clear because the tissue enhances the sounds.

Nursing process step: Assessment

Client needs category: Physiological integrity

Client needs subcategory: Physiological adaptation

Cognitive level: Application

4. A client comes to the emergency department with status asthmaticus. His respiratory rate is 48 breaths/minute and he is wheezing. An arterial blood gas analysis reveals a pH of 7.52, $PaCO_2$ of 30 mm Hg, PO_2 of 7030 mm Hg, and HCO_3^- of 26 mEq/L. What disorder is indicated by these findings?

_____

ANSWER: Respiratory alkalosis

Rationale: Respiratory alkalosis results from alveolar hyperventilation. It's marked by a decrease in partial pressure of arterial carbon dioxide ($PaCO_2$) to less than 35 mm Hg and an increase in blood pH over 7.45.

Nursing process step: Analysis

Client needs category: Physiological integrity

Client needs subcategory: Physiological adaptation

Cognitive level: Application

---

5. A client with a suspected pulmonary embolus is brought in to the emergency department. She complains of shortness of breath and chest pain. Which other signs and symptoms would support this diagnosis?

Select all that apply:

☐ **A.** Low-grade fever

☐ **B.** Thick green sputum

☐ **C.** Bradycardia

☐ **D.** Frothy sputum

☐ **E.** Tachycardia

☐ **F.** Blood-tinged sputum

ANSWER: A, E, F

Rationale: In addition to pleuritic chest pain and dyspnea, a client with a pulmonary embolus may also present with a low-grade fever, tachycardia, and blood-tinged sputum. Thick green sputum would indicate infection, and frothy sputum would indicate pulmonary edema. A client with a pulmonary embolus is tachycardic (to compensate for decreased oxygen supply), not bradycardic.

Nursing process step: Assessment

Client needs category: Physiological integrity

Client needs subcategory: Physiological adaptation

Cognitive level: Application

6. A client with chronic obstructive pulmonary disease (COPD) is being evaluated for a lung transplant. The nurse performs his initial physical assessment. Which signs and symptoms should the nurse expect to find?

Select all that apply:

☐ **A.** Decreased respiratory rate

☐ **B.** Dyspnea on exertion

☐ **C.** Barrel chest

☐ **D.** Shortened expiratory phase

☐ **E.** Clubbed fingers and toes

☐ **F.** Fever

Answer: B, C, E

Rationale: Typical findings for clients with COPD include dyspnea on exertion, a barrel chest, and clubbed fingers and toes. Clients with COPD are usually tachypneic with a prolonged expiratory phase. Fever is not associated with COPD, unless an infection is also present.

Nursing process step: Assessment

Client needs category: Physiological integrity

Client needs subcategory: Physiological adaptation

Cognitive level: Application

---

7. A client with a wound infection develops septic shock. An arterial blood gas analysis reveals pH of 7.25, $PaCO_2$ of 43 mm Hg, PaO_2 of 72 mm Hg, and HCO_3^- of 18 mEq/L. On the following illustration of the oxyhemoglobin dissociation curve, identify which line would reflect his clinical condition.

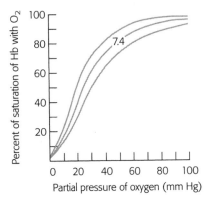

Answer:

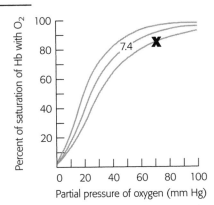

Rationale: The acidic condition of the blood shifts the oxyhemoglobin dissociation curve to the right. This enables oxygen molecules to unload more easily from the hemoglobin.

Nursing process step: Analysis

Client needs category: Physiological integrity

Client needs subcategory: Physiological adaptation

Cognitive level: Analysis

8. A trauma victim in the intensive care unit has a tension pneumothorax. Which of the following signs and symptoms are associated with a tension pneumothorax?

Select all that apply:

☐ **A.** Decreased cardiac output

☐ **B.** Flattened neck veins

☐ **C.** Tracheal deviation to the affected side

☐ **D.** Hypotension

☐ **E.** Tracheal deviation to the opposite side

☐ **F.** Bradypnea

ANSWER: A, D, E

Rationale: Tension pneumothorax results when air in the pleural space is under higher pressure than air in the adjacent lung. The site of the rupture of the pleural space acts as a one-way valve, allowing the air to enter on inspiration but not allowing it to escape on expiration. The air presses against the mediastinum, causing a shift to the opposite side and decreased venous return (reflected by decreased cardiac output and hypotension). This also leads to compensatory tachycardia and tachypnea.

Nursing process step: Assessment

Client needs category: Physiological integrity

Client needs subcategory: Physiological adaptation

Cognitive level: Application

---

9. A client with right middle lobe pneumonia is being cared for in the intensive care unit. In the following illustration of an anterior view of the lungs, identify the area where the nurse may expect to hear associated adventitious breath sounds, such as crackles.

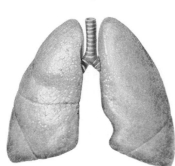

ANSWER:

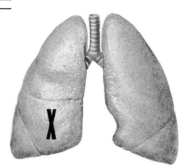

Rationale: The right lung is made up of three lobes: the right upper lobe, right middle lobe, and right lower lobe. The left lung is made up of only two lobes: the left upper lobe and the left lower lobe. When assessing the anterior chest, the right lung is to the examiner's left.

Nursing process step: Assessment

Client needs category: Health promotion and maintenance

Client needs subcategory: Prevention and early detection of disease

Cognitive level: Analysis

10. A client is admitted to the step down unit with an arterial line for continuous measurement of systolic, diastolic, and mean blood pressures. The nurse is evaluating the waveform. Identify the area that indicates that the aortic valve has closed.

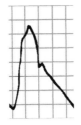

ANSWER:

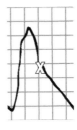

Rationale: When the pressure in the ventricle is less than the pressure in the aortic root, the aortic valve closes. This event appears as a small notch on the waveform's downside.

Nursing process step: Assessment

Client needs category: Physiological integrity

Client needs subcategory: Reduction of risk potential

Cognitive level: Comprehension

---

11. A 33-year-old woman with primary pulmonary hypertension is being evaluated for a heart-lung transplant. The nurse asks her what treatments she is currently receiving for her disease. She is likely to respond by mentioning which treatments?

Select all that apply:

☐ **A.** Oxygen

☐ **B.** Aminoglycosides

☐ **C.** Diuretics

☐ **D.** Vasodilators

☐ **E.** Antihistamines

☐ **F.** Sulfonamides

ANSWER: A, C, D

Rationale: Oxygen, diuretics, and vasodilators are among the common therapies used to treat pulmonary hypertension. Others include fluid restriction, digoxin, calcium channel blockers, beta-adrenergic blockers, and bronchodilators. Aminoglycosides and sulfonamides are antibiotics used to treat infections. Antihistamines are indicated to treat allergy, pruritus, vertigo, nausea, and vomiting; to promote sedation; and to suppress cough.

Nursing process step: Implementation

Client needs category: Physiological integrity

Client needs subcategory: Pharmacological and parenteral therapies

Cognitive level: Application

12. The nurse is performing a respiratory assessment on a client with left lower lobe atelectasis. Identify the area where she may hear fine crackles associated with this condition.

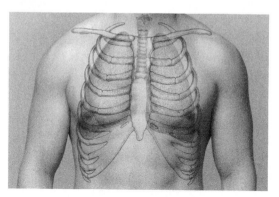

ANSWER:

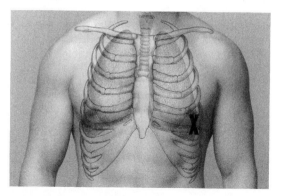

Rationale: To auscultate the left lower lobe from the anterior chest, use the landmarks of the left anterior axillary line, between the fifth and sixth intercostal spaces.

Nursing process step: Assessment

Client needs category: Physiological integrity

Client needs subcategory: Reduction of risk potential

Cognitive level: Application

Genitourinary disorders

1. The nurse is caring for a client diagnosed with acute renal failure. The nurse notes on the intake and output record that the total urine output for the previous 24 hours was 95 ml. What is a urinary output less than 100 ml in 24 hours known as?

ANSWER: Anuria

Rationale: Urine output less than 100 ml in 24 hours is called anuria. Urine output of less than 400 ml but more than 100 ml in 24 hours is called oliguria.

Nursing process step: Implementation

Client needs category: Physiological integrity

Client needs subcategory: Physiological adaptation

Cognitive level: Comprehension

2. A female client reports to the nurse that she experiences a loss of urine when she jogs. The nurse's assessment reveals no nocturia, burning, discomfort when voiding, or urine leakage before reaching the bathroom. The nurse explains to the client that this type of incontinence is called what?

_____

ANSWER: Stress incontinence

Rationale: Stress incontinence is a small loss of urine with activities that increase intra-abdominal pressure, such as running, laughing, sneezing, jumping, coughing, or bending. These symptoms occur only in the daytime.

Nursing process step: Implementation

Client needs category: Physiological integrity

Client needs subcategory: Basic care and comfort

Cognitive level: Application

3. After a retropubic prostatectomy, a client needs continuous bladder irrigation. The client has an I.V. of D_5W infusing at 40 ml/hr and a triple-lumen urinary catheter with normal saline solution infusing at 200 ml/hr. The nurse empties the urinary catheter drainage bag three times during an 8-hour period for a total of 2780 ml. How many milliters does the nurse calculate as urine?

_____

ANSWER: 1180

Rationale: During 8 hours, 1600 ml of bladder irrigation has been infused (200 ml × 8 hr = 1600 ml/8 hr). The nurse then subtracts this amount of infused bladder irrigation from the total volume in the drainage bag (2780 ml − 1600 ml = 1180 ml) to determine urinary output.

Nursing process step: Implementation

Client needs category: Physiological integrity

Client needs subcategory: Basic care and comfort

Cognitive level: Analysis

4. The nurse is caring for a client with chronic renal failure. The laboratory results indicate hypocalcemia and hyperphosphatemia. When assessing the client, the nurse should be alert for which of the following?

Select all that apply:

☐ **A.** Trousseau's sign

☐ **B.** Cardiac arrhythmias

☐ **C.** Constipation

☐ **D.** Decreased clotting time

☐ **E.** Drowsiness and lethargy

☐ **F.** Fractures

ANSWER: A, B, F

Rationale: Hypocalcemia is a calcium deficit that causes nerve fiber irritability and repetitive muscle spasms. Signs and symptoms of hypocalcemia include Trousseau's sign, cardiac arrhythmias, diarrhea, increased clotting times, anxiety, and irritability. The calcium-phosphorus imbalance leads to brittle bones and pathologic fractures.

Nursing process step: Assessment

Client needs category: Physiological integrity

Client needs subcategory: Reduction of risk potential

Cognitive level: Application

---

5. The nurse is assessing a client diagnosed with cystitis. To percuss the kidneys, the nurse locates the costovertebral angle, which is formed by the spinal column and which rib?

ANSWER: 12th

Rationale: Kidney percussion checks for costovertebral angle tenderness that occurs with inflammation. To percuss over the kidneys, have the client sit down and then place the ball of the nondominant hand on the back at the costovertebral angle—the angle formed by the spinal column and the 12th rib. Strike the ball of the hand with the ulnar surface of the other hand and percuss bilaterally.

Nursing process step: Assessment

Client needs category: Physiological integrity

Client needs subcategory: Physiological adaptation

Cognitive level: Application

6. The nurse is caring for a client with acute renal failure. The nurse should expect that hypertonic glucose, insulin infusions, and sodium bicarbonate will be used to treat what complication of acute renal failure?

_____

ANSWER: Hyperkalemia

Rationale: Hyperkalemia is a common complication of acute renal failure. The administration of glucose and regular insulin infusions, with sodium bicarbonate if necessary, can temporarily prevent cardiac arrest by moving potassium into the cells and temporarily reducing potassium levels.

Nursing process step: Planning

Client needs category: Physiological integrity

Client needs subcategory: Pharmacological and parenteral therapies

Cognitive level: Application

Part 3
Maternal-infant nursing

1. A client comes to the office for her first prenatal visit. She reports that January 3 was the first day of her last menstrual period. According to Nägele's rule, what date should the nurse record as the estimated date of delivery (EDD)?

_____

ANSWER: October 10

Rationale: The nurse can calculate EDD using Nägele's rule (add 7 days to the first day of the last menstrual period, then subtract 3 months, and finally add 1 year). In this example, January 3 + 7 days = January 10. 3 months prior to that date is October 10 of the previous year. Adding 1 year, her EDD is October 10 of the current year.

Nursing process step: Analysis

Client needs category: Health promotion and maintenance

Client needs subcategory: Growth and development through the life span

Cognitive level: Application

---

2. A pregnant client at 26 weeks' gestation takes a 1-hour glucose tolerance test as part of a recommended screening for gestational diabetes. A result of greater than or equal to what number of mg/dl indicates the need for further testing?

_____

ANSWER: 140

Rationale: Screening for gestational diabetes using a 1-hour glucose test is recommended for all pregnant women between 24 and 28 weeks' gestation. An abnormal 1-hour glucose tolerance test is defined as a level of 140 mg/dl or greater. A 3-hour standard glucose tolerance test should be performed is results of the 1-hour test are abnormal.

Nursing process step: Analysis

Client needs category: Physiological integrity

Client needs subcategory: Reduction of risk potential

Cognitive level: Application

3. A client who is 14 weeks pregnant states, "Ever since I've been pregnant, I've had a hard time moving my bowels." Increased levels of what hormone are responsible for this common discomfort of pregnancy?

_____

ANSWER: Progesterone

Rationale: Progesterone increases smooth muscle relaxation, thereby decreasing peristalsis. This slowed movement of contents through the GI system can lead to firmer stools and constipation.

Nursing process step: Analysis

Client needs category: Health promotion and maintenance

Client needs subcategory: Growth and development through the life span

Cognitive level: Application

---

4. The nurse is palpating the uterus of a client who is 20 weeks pregnant to measure fundal height. Identify the area on the abdomen where the nurse should expect to feel the uterine fundus.

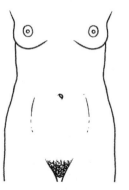

ANSWER:

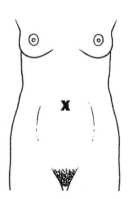

Rationale: At 20 weeks, fundal height should be at approximately the umbilicus. Fundal height should be measured from the symphysis pubis to the top of the uterus. Serial measurements assess fetal growth over the course of the pregnancy. Between weeks 18 and 34, the centimeters measured correlate approximately with the week of gestation.

Nursing process step: Assessment

Client needs category: Health promotion and maintenance

Client needs subcategory: Growth and development through the life span

Cognitive level: Comprehension

5. A client who is 41 weeks pregnant is about to undergo a biophysical profile (BPP) to evaluate her fetus's well-being. The nurse knows that which of the following components are included in a BPP?

Select all that apply:

☐ **A.** Fetal tone

☐ **B.** Fetal breathing movements

☐ **C.** Femur length

☐ **D.** Amniotic fluid volume

☐ **E.** Biparietal diameter

☐ **F.** Crown-rump length

ANSWER: A, B, D

Rationale: The BPP is an ultrasound assessment of the fetus's well-being that includes the following components: nonstress test, fetal tone, fetal breathing, fetal motion, and quantity of amniotic fluid. Crown-rump length is used to assess gestational age and is done during the first trimester. Measurements of the biparietal diameter and femur length are also used to assess gestational age and are done in the second and third trimesters.

Nursing process step: Evaluation

Client needs category: Physiological integrity

Client needs subcategory: Reduction of risk potential

Cognitive level: Application

---

6. The nurse is performing a prenatal assessment on a client who is 32 weeks pregnant. She performs Leopold's maneuvers and determines that the fetus is in the cephalic position. Identify where the nurse should place the Doppler to auscultate fetal heart tones.

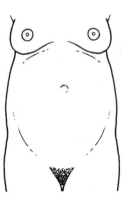

ANSWER:

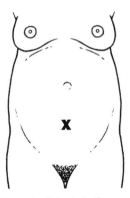

Rationale: When the fetus is in the cephalic position (head down), fetal heart tones are best auscultated midway between the symphysis pubis and the umbilicus. When the fetus is in the breech position, fetal heart tones are best heard at or above the level of the umbilicus.

Nursing process step: Assessment

Client needs category: Health promotion and maintenance

Client needs subcategory: Growth and development through the life span

Cognitive level: Analysis

7. A woman who is 15 weeks pregnant comes to the clinic for amniocentesis. The nurse knows that this test can be used to identify which of the following characteristics or problems?

Select all that apply:

- ☐ **A.** Fetal lung maturity
- ☐ **B.** Gestational diabetes
- ☐ **C.** Chromosomal defects
- ☐ **D.** Neural tube defects
- ☐ **E.** Polyhydramnios
- ☐ **F.** Sex of the fetus

ANSWER: C, D, F

Rationale: In early pregnancy, amniocentesis can identify chromosomal defects and neural tube defects. It can also be used to determine the sex of the fetus. Amniocentesis can be used to evaluate fetal lung maturity only during the last trimester of pregnancy. A blood test performed between 24 and 28 weeks' gestation is used to screen for gestational diabetes. Ultrasound is used to identify polyhydramnios (excessive amount of amniotic fluid); amniocentesis can be used to treat polyhydramnios by removing excess fluid.

Nursing process step: Planning

Client needs category: Physiological integrity

Client needs subcategory: Reduction of risk potential

Cognitive level: Application

---

8. A client who is 32 weeks pregnant is being monitored in the antepartum unit for pregnancy-induced hypertension. She suddenly complains of continuous abdominal pain and vaginal bleeding. Which of the following nursing interventions should be included in the care of this client?

Select all that apply:

- ☐ **A.** Evaluate vital signs.
- ☐ **B.** Prepare for vaginal delivery.
- ☐ **C.** Reassure the client that she'll be able to continue the pregnancy.
- ☐ **D.** Evaluate fetal heart tones.
- ☐ **E.** Monitor the amount of vaginal bleeding.
- ☐ **F.** Monitor intake and output.

ANSWER: A, D, E, F

Rationale: The client's symptoms indicate that she's experiencing abruptio placentae. The nurse must immediately evaluate the mother's well-being by evaluating vital signs; evaluate the well-being of the fetus by auscultating fetal heart tones; monitor the amount of blood loss; and evaluate volume status by monitoring intake and output. After the severity of the abruption has been determined and blood and fluid have been replaced, prompt cesarean delivery of the fetus (not vaginal delivery) is indicated if the fetus is in distress.

Nursing process step: Implementation

Client needs category: Physiological integrity

Client needs subcategory: Physiological adaptation

Cognitive level: Analysis

9. In early pregnancy, some clients complain of abdominal pain or pulling. Identify the area most commonly associated with this pain.

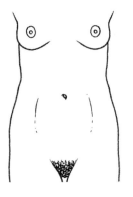

ANSWER:

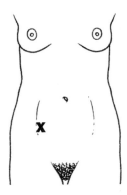

Rationale: As the uterus grows in early pregnancy, it deviates physically to the right. This shift, or dextrorotation, is due to the presence of the rectosigmoid colon in the left lower quadrant. As a result, many women complain of pain in the right lower quadrant.

Nursing process step: Evaluation

Client needs category: Health promotion and maintenance

Client needs subcategory: Growth and development throughout the lifespan

Cognitive level: Analysis

---

10. A woman in her first trimester of pregnancy comes to the prenatal clinic and states, "I feel nauseous and I'm vomiting all the time. I can't even keep down water." This client should be evaluated for what condition?

ANSWER: Hyperemesis gravidarum

Rationale: Hyperemesis gravidarum differs from the nausea and vomiting that normally occur during pregnancy. It's characterized by excessive vomiting that can lead to dehydration and starvation. Without treatment, metabolic changes can lead to severe complications, even death, of the fetus or mother.

Nursing process step: Assessment

Client needs category: Physiological integrity

Client needs subcategory: Physiological adaptation

Cognitive level: Application

11. A pregnant client at 32 weeks' gestation has mild preeclampsia. She is discharged home with instructions to remain on bed rest. She should also be instructed to call her doctor if she experiences which of the following symptoms?

Select all that apply:

☐ **A.** Headache

☐ **B.** Increased urine output

☐ **C.** Blurred vision

☐ **D.** Difficulty sleeping

☐ **E.** Epigastric pain

☐ **F.** Severe nausea and vomiting

ANSWER: A, C, E, F

Rationale: Headache, blurred vision, epigastric pain, and severe nausea and vomiting can indicate worsening maternal disease. Decreased, not increased, urine output is a concern because it could indicate renal impairment. Difficulty sleeping, a common complaint during the third trimester, is only a concern if it's caused by any of the other symptoms.

Nursing process step: Implementation

Client needs category: Physiological integrity

Client needs subcategory: Reduction of risk potential

Cognitive level: Application

---

12. A client who is 37 weeks pregnant comes to the office for a prenatal visit. The nurse performs Leopold's maneuvers to assess the position of the fetus. After performing the maneuvers, the nurse suspects that the physician will attempt external version. Where did the nurse palpate the head of the fetus?

ANSWER:

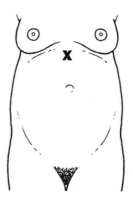

Rationale: If the fetal head is palpated at the top of the uterus, the fetus is in the breech position. That is, the head is not the presenting part and the physician may consider external version to convert the fetus to a vertex lie, or head-down position. This is accomplished by applying pressure on the maternal abdomen to turn the infant over, as in a somersault.

Nursing process step: Planning

Client needs category: Physiological integrity

Client needs subcategory: Reduction of risk potential

Cognitive level: Analysis

13. The nurse is teaching a course on the anatomy and physiology of reproduction. In the illustration of the female reproductive organs, identify the area where fertilization occurs.

ANSWER:

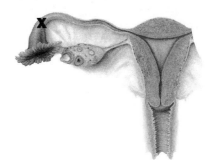

Rationale: After ejaculation, the sperm travel by flagellar movement through the fluids of the cervical mucous into the Fallopian tube to meet the descending ovum in the ampulla. This is where fertilization occurs.

Nursing process step: Implementation

Client needs category: Health promotion and maintenance

Client needs subcategory: Growth and development through the life span

Cognitive level: Application

Intrapartum period

1. The nurse is evaluating a client who is 34 weeks pregnant for premature rupture of the membranes (PROM). Which findings indicate that PROM has occurred?

Select all that apply:

☐ **A.** Fernlike pattern when vaginal fluid is placed on a glass slide and allowed to dry

☐ **B.** Acidic pH of fluid when tested with nitrazine paper

☐ **C.** Presence of amniotic fluid in the vagina

☐ **D.** Cervical dilation of 6 cm

☐ **E.** Alkaline pH of fluid when tested with nitrazine paper

☐ **F.** Contractions occurring every 5 minutes

ANSWER: A, C, E

Rationale: The fernlike pattern that occurs when vaginal fluid is placed on a glass slide and allowed to dry, presence of amniotic fluid in the vagina, and alkaline pH of fluid are all signs of ruptured membranes. The fernlike pattern seen when the fluid is allowed to dry on a slide is a result of the high sodium and protein content of the amniotic fluid. The presence of amniotic fluid in the vagina results from the expulsion of the fluid from the amniotic sac. Cervical dilation and regular contractions are signs of progressing labor but do not indicate PROM.

Nursing process step: Assessment

Client needs category: Physiological integrity

Client needs subcategory: Physiological adaptation

Cognitive level: Analysis

2. A client in the first stage of labor is being monitored using an external fetal monitor. The nurse notes variable decelerations on the monitoring strip. Into what position should the nurse assist the client?

_____

ANSWER: Left lateral
_____

Rationale: Variable decelerations are transient drops in the fetal heart rate that can occur before, during, or after a contraction. The left lateral position is the ideal position for any pregnant client, as it prevents maternal hypotension caused by inferior vena cava compression, which reduces placental perfusion.

Nursing process step: Implementation

Client needs category: Physiological integrity

Client needs subcategory: Reduction of risk potential

Cognitive level: Analysis

---

3. On the waveform below, identify the area that indicates possible umbilical cord compression.

_____

ANSWER:
_____

Rationale: Variable decelerations are decreases in fetal heart rate that aren't related to the timing of contractions. Characteristic of umbilical cord compression, variable decelerations generally occur as drops of 10 to 60 beats/minute below the baseline.

Nursing process step: Assessment

Client needs category: Physiological integrity

Client needs subcategory: Reduction of risk potential

Cognitive level: Analysis

4. A client who is 29 weeks pregnant comes to the labor and delivery unit. She states that she's having contractions every 8 minutes. The client is also 3 cm dilated. Which of the following can the nurse expect to administer?

Select all that apply:

☐ **A.** Folic acid (Folvite)

☐ **B.** Terbutaline (Brethine)

☐ **C.** Betamethasone

☐ **D.** Rh$_o$ (D) immune globulin (Rhogam)

☐ **E.** I.V. fluids

☐ **F.** Meperidine (Demerol)

ANSWER: B, C, E

Rationale: The client is at risk for preterm delivery. The nurse can expect that terbutaline, a beta-2 agonist that relaxes smooth muscle, will be administered to halt contractions. The nurse can also expect that betamethasone, a corticosteroid, will be administered to decrease the risk of respiratory distress in the infant if preterm delivery occurs and I.V. fluids will be used to expand the intravascular volume and decrease contractions, if dehydration is the cause. Folic acid is a mineral recommended throughout pregnancy (especially in the first trimester) to decrease the risk of neural tube defects. It isn't used to address preterm delivery. Rh$_o$ (D) immune globulin is administered to Rh-negative clients who have been or are suspected of having been exposed to Rh-positive fetal blood. Meperidine is a narcotic used during labor and delivery to manage pain.

Nursing process step: Implementation

Client needs category: Physiological integrity

Client needs subcategory: Pharmacological and parenteral therapies

Cognitive level: Analysis

---

5. The nurse is monitoring a client who is receiving oxytocin (Pitocin) to induce labor. The nurse should be prepared for which of the following maternal adverse reactions?

Select all that apply:

☐ **A.** Hypertension

☐ **B.** Jaundice

☐ **C.** Dehydration

☐ **D.** Fluid overload

☐ **E.** Uterine tetany

☐ **F.** Bradycardia

ANSWER: A, D, E

Rationale: Adverse reactions to oxytocin in the mother include hypertension, fluid overload, and uterine tetany. The antidiuretic effect of oxytocin increases renal reabsorption of water, leading to fluid overload — not dehydration. Jaundice and bradycardia are adverse reactions that may occur in the neonate. Tachycardia, not bradycardia, is reported as a maternal adverse reaction.

Nursing process step: Planning

Client needs category: Physiological integrity

Client needs subcategory: Pharmacological and parenteral therapies

Cognitive level: Application

6. The nurse is evaluating the external fetal monitoring strip of a client who is in labor. She notes decreases in the fetal heart rate (FHR) that coincide with the client's contractions. What term does the nurse use to document this finding?

_____

ANSWER: Early decelerations

Rationale: A deceleration is a decrease in the FHR below the baseline. When decelerations occur at the same time as uterine contractions, they're called *early decelerations.* Early decelerations result from head compression during normal labor and do not indicate fetal distress.

Nursing process step: Analysis

Client needs category: Health promotion and maintenance

Client needs subcategory: Growth and development through the life span

Cognitive level: Application

---

7. A client in labor is 8 cm dilated. The fetus, which is in vertex presentation, is 75% effaced and is at 0 station. In the illustration below, identify the level of the fetus's head.

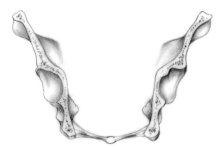

ANSWER:

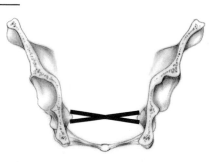

Rationale: Station refers to the level of the presenting part in relation to the pelvic inlet and the ischial spines. A 0 station indicates that the presenting part lies at the level of the ischial spines. Other stations are defined by their distance in centimeters above or below the ischial spines.

Nursing process step: Assessment

Client needs category: Health promotion and maintenance

Client needs subcategory: Growth and development through the life span

Cognitive level: Application

8. The nurse is evaluating an external fetal monitoring strip. Identify the area on this strip that causes her to be concerned about uteroplacental insufficiency.

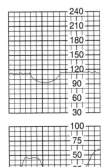

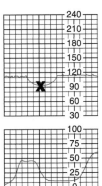

Rationale: This fetal monitoring strip illustrates a late deceleration. The decrease in fetal heart rate begins at the end of the contraction and does not return to baseline until the contraction is over. Late decelerations are associated with uteroplacental insufficiency, shock, or fetal metabolic acidosis.

Nursing process step: Assessment

Client needs category: Physiological integrity

Client needs subcategory: Reduction of risk potential

Cognitive level: Analysis

---

9. A client with diabetes gives birth to a 9-lb, 10-oz neonate at 38 weeks. Which of the neonate's serum level should be assessed immediately after birth?

ANSWER: Glucose

Rationale: Glucose monitoring of the infant born to a mother with diabetes is essential because he is at risk for developing hypoglycemia after birth.

Nursing process step: Evaluation

Client needs category: Physiological integrity

Client needs subcategory: Reduction of risk potential

Cognitive level: Application

10. The nurse is evaluating a fetal monitoring strip to time the contractions of a laboring client. Identify the beginning of the contraction in the illustration below.

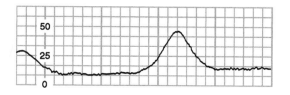

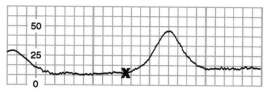

Rationale: The beginning of a contraction, identified by a rise in pressure in the uterus, is indicated on the monitoring strip by movement of the waveform away from the baseline.

Nursing process step: Assessment

Client needs category: Health promotion and maintenance

Client needs subcategory: Growth and development through the life span

Cognitive level: Application

Postpartum period

1. The nurse is instructing a client about breast-feeding. Which instructions should she include to help prevent the mother from developing mastitis?

Select all that apply:

☐ **A.** Wash the nipples with soap and water.

☐ **B.** Change the breast pads frequently.

☐ **C.** Expose the nipples to air for part of each day.

☐ **D.** Wash hands before handling the breast and breast-feeding.

☐ **E.** Make sure that the baby grasps the nipple only.

☐ **F.** Release the baby's grasp on the nipple before removing the baby from the breast.

ANSWER: B, C, D, F

Rationale: Because mastitis is an infection frequently associated with a break in the skin surface of the nipple, measures to prevent cracked and fissured nipples help prevent mastitis. Changing breast pads frequently and exposing the nipples to air for part of the day help keep the nipples dry and prevent irritation. Washing hands before handling the breast reduces the chance of accidentally introducing organisms into the breast. Releasing the baby's grasp on the nipple before removing the baby from the breast also reduces the chance of irritation. Nipples should be washed with water only; soap tends to remove the natural oils and increases the chance of cracking. The baby should grasp both the nipple and areola.

Nursing process step: Planning

Client needs category: Health promotion and maintenance

Client needs subcategory: Prevention and early detection of disease

Cognitive level: Comprehension

2. The nurse is caring for a 1-day postpartum mother who's very talkative but isn't confident in her decision-making skills. The nurse is aware that this is a normal phase for the mother. What is this phase called?

_____

Rationale: The taking-in phase is a normal first phase for a mother when she's feeling overwhelmed by the responsibilities of newborn care, while still fatigued from delivery. Taking hold is the next phase, when the mother has rested and she can think and learn mothering skills with confidence.

Nursing process step: Assessment

Client needs category: Psychosocial integrity

Client needs subcategory: Psychosocial adaptation

Cognitive level: Analysis

---

3. The nurse observes several interactions between a mother and her neonate son. Which of the following behaviors of the mother would the nurse identify as evidence of mother-infant attachment?

Select all that apply:

☐ **A.** Talks and coos to her son.

☐ **B.** Cuddles her son close to her.

☐ **C.** Doesn't make eye contact with her son.

☐ **D.** Requests that the nurse take the baby to the nursery for feedings.

☐ **E.** Encourages the father to hold the baby.

☐ **G** Takes a nap when the baby is sleeping.

ANSWER: **A, B**

Rationale: Talking, cooing, and cuddling with her son are positive signs that the mother is adapting to her new role as mother. Avoiding eye contact is a non-bonding behavior. Eye contact, touching, and speaking help establish attachment with a neonate. Feeding a neonate is an important role of a new mother and facilitates attachment. Encouraging the father to hold the neonate will facilitate attachment between the neonate and his father. Resting while the neonate is sleeping will conserve needed energy and allow the mother to be alert and awake when her infant is awake; however it isn't evidence of bonding.

Nursing process step: Evaluation

Client needs category: Psychosocial integrity

Client needs subcategory: Psychosocial adaptation

Cognitive level: Analysis

4. The nurse is caring for a postpartum mother suspected of developing postpartum psychosis. Which of the following statements accurately characterize this disorder?

Select all that apply:

☐ **A.** Symptoms start 2 days after delivery.

☐ **B.** The disorder is common in postpartum women.

☐ **C.** Symptoms include delusions and hallucinations.

☐ **D.** Suicide and infanticide are uncommon in this disorder.

☐ **E.** The disorder rarely occurs without psychiatric history.

ANSWER: C, E

Rationale: A postpartum woman should be suspected of psychosis if she exhibits manic-depressive behaviors (delusions or hallucinations), generally starting within 4 weeks postpartum. Typically, the woman has a past history of a psychiatric disorder and treatment. The disorder occurs in less then 1% of postpartum mothers. It's considered a medical emergency. Suicide and infanticide are common.

Nursing process step: Assessment

Client needs category: Psychosocial integrity

Client needs subcategory: Psychosocial adaptation

Cognitive level: Analysis

---

5. A mother with a past history of varicose veins has just delivered her first baby. The nurse suspects that the mother has developed a pulmonary embolus. Which of the data below would lead to this nursing judgment?

Select all that apply:

☐ **A.** Sudden dyspnea

☐ **B.** Chills, fever

☐ **C.** Diaphoresis

☐ **D.** Hypertension

☐ **E.** Confusion

ANSWER: A, C, E

Rationale: Sudden dyspnea with diaphoresis and confusion are classic signs and symptoms of dislodgment of a thrombus (stationary blood clot) from a varicose vein becoming an embolus (moving clot) that lodges itself into the pulmonary circulation. Chills and fever would indicate an infection. A client with an embolus could be hypotensive, not hypertensive.

Nursing process step: Assessment

Client needs category: Physiological integrity

Client needs subcategory: Physiological adaptation

Cognitive level: Analysis

6. The nurse is palpating the uterine fundus of a client who delivered a baby 8 hours ago. At what level in the abdomen would the nurse expect to feel the fundus?

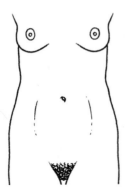

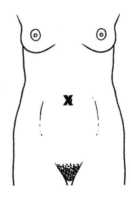

Rationale: The uterus should be felt at the level of the umbilicus from 1 hour after birth and for approximately the next 24 hours.

Nursing process step: Assessment

Client needs category: Physiological integrity

Client needs subcategory: Reduction of risk potential

Cognitive level: Comprehension

---

7. In the fourth stage of labor, a full bladder increases the risk of what postpartum complication?

ANSWER: Hemorrhage

Rationale: A full bladder prevents the uterus from contracting completely, increasing the risk of hemorrhage.

Nursing process step: Assessment

Client needs category: Physiological integrity

Client needs subcategory: Reduction of risk potential

Cognitive level: Knowledge

8. On a client's first postpartum day, the nurse assesses the client's vaginal discharge as dark red and containing shreds of decidua and mucus. What term should the nurse use in her nurse's notes to describe the discharge?

_____

ANSWER: Lochia rubra

Rationale: For the first 3 days after birth, a lochia discharge consists almost entirely of blood with only small particles of decidua and mucus. Because of its red color, it's called *lochia rubra*.

Nursing process step: Assessment

Client needs category: Physiological integrity

Client needs subcategory: Physiological adaptation

Cognitive level: Knowledge

---

9. The nurse is providing teaching to a postpartum client who has decided to breast-feed her neonate. She has questions regarding her nutritional intake and wants to know how many extra calories she should eat. What number of additional calories should the nurse instruct the client to eat per day?

_____

ANSWER: 500

Rationale: The recommended energy intake for a lactating mother is 500 kcal more than their nonpregnant intake.

Nursing process step: Implementation

Client needs category: Health promotion and maintenance

Client needs subcategory: Growth and development through the life span

Cognitive level: Application

The neonate

1. The nurse is doing a neurologic assessment on a 1-day-old neonate in the nursery. Which of the following findings would indicate possible asphyxia in utero?

Select all that apply:

- ☐ **A.** The neonate grasps the nurse's finger when she puts it in the palm of his hand.
- ☐ **B.** The neonate does stepping movements when held upright with sole of foot touching a surface.
- ☐ **C.** The neonate's toes don't curl downward when soles of feet are stroked.
- ☐ **D.** The neonate doesn't respond when the nurse claps her hands above him.
- ☐ **E.** The neonate turns toward the nurse's finger when she touches his cheek.
- ☐ **F.** The neonate displays weak, ineffective sucking.

ANSWER: C, D, F

Rationale: If the neonate's toes don't curl downward when the soles of his feet are stroked and he doesn't respond to a loud sound, it may be evidence that neurologic damage from asphyxia has occurred. A normal neurologic response would be the toes curling downward with stroking and extending arms and legs with a loud noise. Weak, ineffective sucking is another sign of neurologic damage. A neonate should grasp a person's finger when it's placed in the palm of his hand, do stepping movements when held upright with the sole of foot touching a surface, and turn toward the nurse's finger when she touches his cheek.

Nursing process step: Assessment

Client needs category: Health promotion and maintenance

Client needs subcategory: Growth and development through the life span

Cognitive level: Application

---

2. What information should the nurse include when teaching postcircumcision care to parents of a neonate prior to discharge from the hospital?

Select all that apply:

- ☐ **A.** The infant must void before being discharged home.
- ☐ **B.** Petroleum jelly should be applied to the glans of the penis with each diaper change.
- ☐ **C.** The infant can take tub baths while the circumcision heals.
- ☐ **D.** Any blood noted on the front of the diaper should be reported.
- ☐ **E.** The circumcision will require care for 2 to 4 days after discharge.

ANSWER: A, B, E

Rationale: It's necessary for the infant to void prior to discharge to ensure that the urethra isn't obstructed. A lubricating ointment is appropriate and is applied with each diaper change. Typically, the penis heals within 2 to 4 days, and circumcision care is needed for that period only. To prevent infection, avoid giving the infant tub baths until the circumcision is healed; sponge baths are appropriate. A small amount of bleeding is expected following a circumcision; parents should report only a large amount of bleeding.

Nursing process step: Implementation

Client needs category: Safe, effective care environment

Client needs subcategory: Management of care

Cognitive level: Application

3. A 14-day-old neonate is admitted for aspiration pneumonia. The results of a barium swallow confirm a diagnosis of gastroesophageal reflux with resulting aspiration pneumonia. Identify the area of the stomach that is weakened, and thus contributing to the reflux.

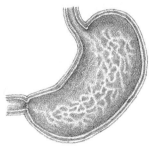

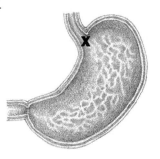

Rationale: Gastroesophageal reflux is a neuromotor disturbance in which the cardiac sphincter located between the stomach and the esophagus is lax. This allows easy regurgitation of gastric contents into the esophagus, causing possible aspiration into the lungs.

Nursing process step: Analysis

Client needs category: Physiological integrity

Client needs subcategory: Physiological adaptation

Cognitive level: Comprehension

---

4. A nurse is demonstrating cord care to a mother of a neonate. Which actions would the nurse teach the mother to perform?

Select all that apply:

☐ **A.** Keep the diaper below the cord.

☐ **B.** Tug gently on the cord as it begins to dry.

☐ **C.** Apply antibiotic ointment to the cord twice daily.

☐ **D.** Only sponge-bathe the infant until the cord falls off.

☐ **E.** Clean the length of the cord with alcohol several times daily.

☐ **F.** Wash the cord with mild soap and water.

ANSWER: A, D, E

Rationale: The diaper should be positioned below the cord to allow it to air dry and to prevent urine from getting on the cord. Soap and water should not be used as a part of cord care. The nurse should instruct the parents to sponge bathe the infant until the cord falls off. The entire cord should be cleaned with alcohol, using a cotton swab or another appropriate method. Parents should also be instructed to never pull on the cord, but to allow it to fall off naturally. Antibiotic ointments are contraindicated unless there are signs of infection.

Nursing process step: Implementation

Client needs category: Safe, effective care

Client needs subcategory: Safety and infection control

Cognitive level: Application

5. At 5 minutes of age, a neonate is pink with acrocyanosis, has his knees flexed and fists clinched, has a whimpering cry, has a heart rate of 128, and withdraws his foot when slapped on the sole. What 5-minute Apgar score would the nurse record for this neonate?

Sign	Apgar Score		
	0	1	2
Heart rate	Absent	Less than 100 beats/ minute (slow)	More than 100 beats/ minute
Respiratory effort	Absent	Slow, irregular	Good crying
Muscle tone	Flaccid	Some flexion and resistance to extension of extremities	Active motion
Reflex irritability	No response	Grimace or weak cry	Vigorous cry
Color	Pallor, cyanosis	Pink body, blue extremities	Completely pink

ANSWER: 8

Rationale: Apgar consists of a 0 to 2 point scoring system for a neonate immediately following birth and at 5 minutes of age. The nurse evaluates the neonate for heart rate, respiratory effort, muscle tone, reflex irritability, and color. This neonate has a heart rate above 100, which equals 2; pink color with acrocyanosis, which equals 1; is well-flexed, which equals 2; has a weak cry, which equals 1; and has a good response to slapping the soles of the feet, which equals 2. Therefore, the nurse should record a total Apgar score of 8.

Nursing process step: Assessment

Client needs category: Physiological integrity

Client needs subcategory: Physiological adaptation

Cognitive level: Analysis

6. A nurse is conducting a physical examination on a neonate. At which pulse point on an infant would the absence of a palpable pulse indicate a possible coarctation of the aorta?

ANSWER: Femoral

Rationale: With coarctation of the aorta, the nurse should note bounding pulses and increased blood pressure in the upper extremities, as well as decreased or absent pulses and lower blood pressure in the lower extremities. This is due to the narrowing of the aortic arch.

Nursing process step: Assessment

Client needs category: Physiological integrity

Client needs subcategory: Physiological adaptation

Cognitive level: Application

7. A nurse is administering vitamin K (AquaMEPHY-TON) to a neonate following delivery. The medication comes in a concentration of 2 mg/ml and the ordered dose is 0.5 mg to be given subcutaneously. How many milliliters should the nurse administer?

_____

ANSWER: 0.25

Rationale: Use the following formula to calculate drug dosages:

Dose on hand/Quantity on hand = Dose desired/X

Plug in the values and the equation is as follows:

$$2 \text{ mg/ml} = 0.5 \text{ mg/X;}$$

$$X = 0.25 \text{ ml}$$

Nursing process step: Analysis

Client needs category: Physiological integrity

Client needs subcategory: Pharmacological and parenteral therapies

Cognitive level: Analysis

---

8. A nurse is eliciting reflexes in a neonate during a physical examination. Identify the area the nurse would touch to elicit a plantar grasp reflex.

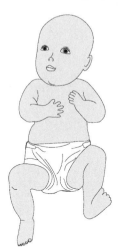

ANSWER:

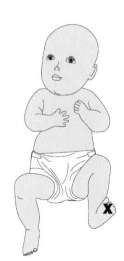

Rationale: To elicit a plantar grasp reflex, the nurse should touch the sole of the foot near the base of the digits, causing flexion or grasping. This reflex disappears around age 9 months.

Nursing process step: Assessment

Client needs category: Health promotion and maintenance

Client needs subcategory: Growth and development through the life span

Cognitive level: Application

Part 4
Pediatric nursing

1. The physician orders an I.V. infusion of dextrose 5% in quarter-normal saline solution to be infused at 7 ml/kg/hour for a 10-month-old infant. The infant weighs 22 lb. How many ml/hr should the nurse infuse of the ordered solution?

_____

ANSWER: 70

_____

Rationale: To perform this dosage calculation, the nurse should first convert the infant's weight to kilograms:

$$2.2 \text{ lb/kg} = 22 \text{ lb/X kg}$$

$$X = 22 \div 2.2$$

$$X = 10 \text{ kg}$$

Next, she should multiply the infant's weight by the ordered rate:

$$10 \text{ kg} \times 7 \text{ ml/kg/hr} = 70 \text{ ml/hr}$$

Nursing process step: Implementation

Client needs category: Physiological integrity

Client needs subcategory: Pharmacological and parenteral therapies

Cognitive level: Application

---

2. The nurse is teaching the parents of a 6-month-old infant about usual growth and development. Which of the following statements is true regarding infant development?

Select all that apply:

☐ **A.** A 6-month-old infant has difficulty holding objects.

☐ **B.** A 6-month-old infant can usually roll from prone to supine and supine to prone positions.

☐ **C.** A teething ring is appropriate for a 6-month-old infant.

☐ **D.** Stranger anxiety usually peaks at age 12 to 18 months.

☐ **E.** Head lag is commonly noted in infants at age 6 months.

☐ **F.** Lack of visual coordination usually resolves by age 6 months.

ANSWER: B, C, F

_____

Rationale: Gross motor skills of the 6-month-old infant include rolling from front to back and back to front. Teething usually begins around age 6 months and, therefore, a teething ring is appropriate. Visual coordination is usually resolved by age 6 months. At age 6 months, fine motor skills include purposeful grasps. Stranger anxiety normally peaks at 8 months of age. The 6-month-old infant also should have good head control and no longer display head lag when pulled up to a sitting position.

Nursing process step: Implementation

Client needs category: Health promotion and maintenance

Client needs subcategory: Growth and development through the life span

Cognitive level: Application

3. An infant who weighs 7.5 kg is to receive ampicillin (Omnipen) 25 mg/kg I.V. every 6 hours. How many milligrams should the nurse administer per dose?

Rationale: The nurse should calculate the correct dose using the following equation:

$$25 \text{ mg/kg} \times 7.5 \text{ kg} = 187.5 \text{ mg}$$

Nursing process step: Implementation

Client needs category: Physiologic integrity

Client needs subcategory: Pharmacological and parenteral therapies

Cognitive level: Application

---

4. A nurse is conducting a physical examination on an infant. Identify the anatomical landmark she should use to measure chest circumference.

ANSWER:

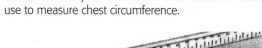

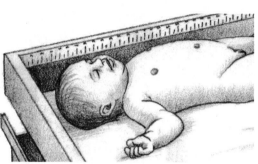

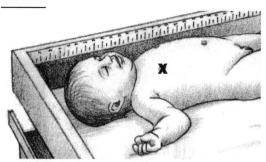

Rationale: Chest circumference is most accurately measured by placing the measuring tape around the infant's chest with the tape covering the nipples. If measured above or below the nipples, a false measurement is obtained.

Nursing process step: Assessment

Client needs category: Health promotion and maintenance

Client needs subcategory: Prevention and early detection of disease

Cognitive level: Application

5. A healthy 2-month-old infant is being seen in the local clinic for a well-child check-up and his initial immunizations. The nurse should anticipate administering which immunizations?

Select all that apply:

☐ **A.** DTaP (diphtheria, tetanus, and acellular pertussis)

☐ **B.** MMR (measles, mumps, and rubella)

☐ **C.** OPV (oral polio vaccine)

☐ **D.** HBV (hepatitis B vaccine)

☐ **E.** Varicella (chicken pox) vaccine

☐ **F.** HIB (Haemophilus influenzae vaccine)

ANSWER: A, D, F

Rationale: At age 2 months, the American Academy of Pediatrics recommends the administration of DTaP, IPV (inactivated polio vaccine), HBV, and HIB. The MMR immunization should be administered at 12 to 15 months. The IPV—not the OPV—is currently used to minimize spread of the disease. Infants may receive the varicella vaccine any time after the child's first birthday.

Nursing process step: Implementation

Client needs category: Health promotion and maintenance

Client needs subcategory: Prevention and early detection of disease

Cognitive level: Application

---

6. When assessing an infant for changes in intracranial pressure (ICP), it's important to palpate the fontanels. Identify the area where the nurse should palpate to assess the anterior fontanel.

ANSWER:

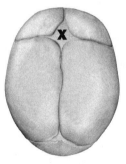

Rationale: The anterior fontanel is formed by the junction of the sagittal, frontal, and coronal sutures. It's shaped like a diamond and normally measures 4 to 5 cm at its widest point. A widened, bulging fontanel is a sign of increased ICP.

Nursing process step: Assessment

Client needs category: Health promotion and maintenance

Client needs subcategory: Prevention and early detection of disease

Cognitive level: Application

7. A parent is planning to enroll her 9-month-old infant in a daycare facility. The parent asks the nurse what to look for as indicators that the daycare facility is adhering to good infection control measures. How should the nurse reply?

Select all that apply:

☐ **A.** The facility keeps boxes of gloves in the director's office.

☐ **B.** Diapers are discarded into covered receptacles.

☐ **C.** Toys are kept on the floor for the children to share.

☐ **D.** Disposable papers are used on the diaper-changing surfaces.

☐ **E.** Facilities for handwashing are located in every classroom.

☐ **F.** Soiled clothing and cloth diapers are sent home in labeled paper bags.

ANSWER: B, D, E

Rationale: A parent can assess infection control measures by appraising steps taken by the facility to prevent the spread of potential diseases. Placing diapers in covered receptacles, covering the diaper-changing surfaces with disposable papers, and ensuring that there are available sinks for personnel to wash their hands after activities are all indicators that infection control measures are being followed. Gloves should be readily available to personnel and, therefore, should be kept in every room — not in an office. Toys typically are shared by numerous children; however, this contributes to the spread of germs and infections. All soiled clothing and cloth diapers should be placed in a sealed plastic bag prior to being sent home.

Nursing process step: Implementation

Client needs category: Safe, effective care environment

Client needs subcategory: Safety and infection control

Cognitive level: Application

---

8. A nurse is performing cardiopulmonary resuscitation on (CPR) an infant. Identify the area where the nurse should assess for a pulse.

ANSWER:

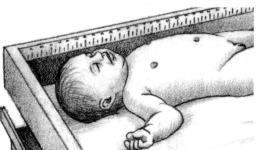

Rationale: The brachial pulse should be used to assess for a pulse when performing infant CPR. The carotid pulse, which is used in children and adults, is extremely difficult to locate in an infant because of his short neck.

Nursing process step: Assessment

Client needs category: Physiological adaptation

Client needs subcategory: Physiological integrity

Cognitive level: Application

9. An infant is having his 2-month checkup at the pediatrician's office. The physician tells the parents that she's assessing for Ortolani's sign. The nurse explains that this is to assess for dislocation of what joint?

_____

ANSWER: Hip

Rationale: To assess for Ortolani's sign the nurse abducts the infant's hips while flexing the legs at the knees. This is performed on all infants to assess for congenital hip dislocation. The examiner listens and feels for a "click" as the femoral head enters the acetabulum during the examination. This finding indicates a congenitally dislocated hip.

Nursing process step: Implementation

Client needs category: Health promotion and maintenance

Client needs subcategory: Prevention and early detection of disease

Cognitive level: Analysis

---

10. A nurse is conducting an infant nutrition class for parents. Which of the following foods should the nurse tell parents it's okay to introduce during the first year of life?

Select all that apply:

☐ **A.** Sliced beef

☐ **B.** Pureed fruits

☐ **C.** Whole milk

☐ **D.** Rice cereal

☐ **E.** Strained vegetables

☐ **F.** Fruit juice

ANSWER: B, D, E

Rationale: The first food provided to a neonate is breast milk or formula. Between ages 4 and 6 months, rice cereal can be introduced, followed by pureed or strained fruits and vegetables, then strained or ground meat. Meats must be chopped or ground prior to feeding them to an infant to prevent choking. Infants should not be given whole milk until they are at least 1 year old. Fruit drinks provide no nutritional benefit and shouldn't be encouraged.

Nursing process step: Implementation

Client needs category: Health promotion and maintenance

Client needs subcategory: Growth and development through the life span

Cognitive level: Application

1. The nurse is preparing a dose of amoxicillin for a 3-year-old with acute otitis media. The child weighs 33 lb. The dosage prescribed is 50 mg/kg/day in divided doses every 8 hours. The concentration of the drug is 250 mg/5 ml. How many milliliters should the nurse administer?

ANSWER: 5

Rationale: To calculate the child's weight in kilograms, the nurse should use the following formula:

$$2.2 \text{ lb}/1 \text{ kg} = 33 \text{ lb}/X \text{ kg}$$

$$X = 33 \div 2.2$$

$$X = 15 \text{ kg}$$

Next, the nurse should calculate the daily dosage for the child:

$$50 \text{ mg/kg/day} \times 15 \text{ kg} = 750 \text{ mg/day}$$

To determine divided daily dosage, the nurse should know that "every 8 hours" means 3 times per day. So, she should perform that calculation in this way:

$$\text{Total daily dosage} \div 3 \text{ times per day} = \text{Divided daily dosage}$$

$$750 \text{ mg/day} \div 3 = 250 \text{ mg}$$

The drug's concentration is 250 mg/5 ml, so the nurse should administer 5 ml.

Nursing process step: Implementation

Client needs category: Physiological integrity

Client needs subcategory: Pharmacological and parenteral therapies

Cognitive level: Application

2. A 3-year-old is to receive 500 ml of dextrose 5% in normal saline solution over 8 hours. At what rate (in ml/hr) should the nurse set the infusion pump?

ANSWER: 62.5

Rationale: To calculate the rate per hour for the infusion, the nurse should divide 500 ml by 8 hours:

$$500 \text{ ml} \div 8 \text{ hours} = 62.5 \text{ ml/hr.}$$

Nursing process step: Implementation

Client needs category: Physiological integrity

Client needs subcategory: Pharmacological and parenteral therapies

Cognitive level: Application

3. A 2½-year-old is being treated for left lower lobe pneumonia. In what position should the nurse position the toddler to maximize oxygenation?

_____

ANSWER: Right lateral

Rationale: The toddler should be positioned on his right side. Gravity contributes to increased blood flow to the right lung, thereby allowing for better gas exchange.

Nursing process step: Implementation

Client needs category: Physiological integrity

Client needs subcategory: Physiological adaptation

Cognitive level: Analysis

---

4. A nurse is feeling the apical impulse of a 28-month-old child. Identify the area where the nurse should assess the apical impulse.

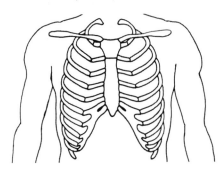

ANSWER:

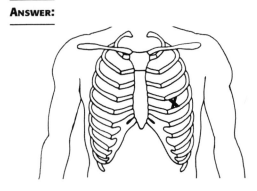

Rationale: The heart's apex for a toddler is located at the fourth intercostal space immediately to the left of the midclavicular line. It's one or two intercostal spaces above what's considered normal for the adult because the heart's position in a child of this age is more horizontal and larger in diameter than that of an adult.

Nursing process step: Assessment

Client needs category: Health promotion and maintenance

Client needs subcategory: Prevention and early detection of disease

Cognitive level: Application

5. A 15-month-old has just received his routine immunizations, including diphtheria, tetanus, and acellular pertussis (DTaP); inactivated polio vaccine (IPV); and measles, mumps, and rubella (MMR). What information should the nurse give to the parents before they leave the office?

Select all that apply:

- ☐ **A.** Minor symptoms can be treated with acetaminophen (Tylenol).
- ☐ **B.** Minor symptoms can be treated with aspirin (A.S.A.).
- ☐ **C.** Call the office if the toddler develops a fever above 103° F (39.4° C), seizures, or difficulty breathing.
- ☐ **D.** Soreness at the immunization site and mild fever are common.
- ☐ **E.** The immunizations prevent the toddler from contracting their associated diseases.
- ☐ **F.** The toddler should restrict his activity for the remainder of the day.

ANSWER: A, C, D

Rationale: Minor symptoms, such as soreness at the immunization site and mild fever, can be treated with acetaminophen or ibuprofen. Aspirin should be avoided in children because of its association with Reye's syndrome. The parents should notify the clinic if serious complications (such as a fever above 103° F, seizures, or difficulty breathing) occur. Minor discomforts, such as soreness and mild fever, are common after immunizations. Immunizing the child decreases the health risks associated with contracting certain diseases; it doesn't prevent the toddler from acquiring them. Although the child may prefer to rest after immunizations, it isn't necessary to restrict his activity.

Nursing process step: Implementation

Client needs category: Health promotion and maintenance

Client needs subcategory: Prevention and early detection of disease

Cognitive level: Application

---

6. A 2-year-old boy is brought into the clinic with an upper respiratory infection. During the assessment, the nurse notes some bruising on the arms, legs, and trunk. Which findings would prompt the nurse to evaluate for suspected child abuse?

Select all that apply:

- ☐ **A.** A few superficial scrapes on the lower legs
- ☐ **B.** Welts or bruises in various stages of healing on the trunk
- ☐ **C.** A deep blue-black patch on the buttocks
- ☐ **D.** One large bruise on the child's thigh
- ☐ **E.** Circular, symmetrical burns on the lower legs
- ☐ **F.** A parent who is hypercritical of the child and pushes the frightened child away

ANSWER: B, E, F

Rationale: Injuries at various stages of healing in protected or padded areas can be signs of inflicted trauma, leading the nurse to suspect abuse. Burns that are bilateral as well as symmetrical and regular are typical of child abuse. The shape of the burn may resemble the item used to create it, such as a cigarette. When a child is burned accidentally, the burns form an erratic pattern and are usually irregular or asymmetrical. Pushing away the child and being hypercritical are typical behaviors of abusive parents. Superficial scrapes and bruises on the lower extremities are normal in a healthy active child. A deep blue-black macular patch on the buttocks is more consistent with a Mongolian spot rather than a traumatic injury that would suggest abuse.

Nursing process step: Analysis

Client needs category: Psychosocial integrity

Client needs subcategory: Psychosocial adaptation

Cognitive level: Analysis

7. A nurse is caring for a 3-year-old with viral meningitis. Which signs and symptoms would the nurse expect to find during the initial assessment?

Select all that apply:

☐ **A.** Bulging anterior fontanel

☐ **B.** Fever

☐ **C.** Nuchal rigidity

☐ **D.** Petechiae

☐ **E.** Irritability

☐ **F.** Photophobia

☐ **G.** Hypothermia

ANSWER: B, C, E, F

Rationale: Common signs and symptoms of viral meningitis include fever, nuchal rigidity, irritability, and photophobia. A bulging anterior fontanel is a sign of hydrocephalus, which isn't likely to occur in a toddler because the anterior fontanel typically closes by age 24 months. A petechial, purpuric rash may be seen with bacterial meningitis. Hypothermia is a common sign of bacterial meningitis in an infant younger than age 3 months.

Nursing process step: Assessment

Client needs category: Physiological integrity

Client needs subcategory: Physiological adaptation

Cognitive level: Application

---

8. A 30-month-old toddler is being evaluated for a ventricular septal defect (VSD). Identify the area where a VSD occurs.

ANSWER:

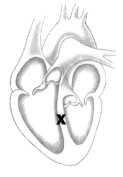

Rationale: A VSD is a small hole between the right and left ventricles. It's a common congenital heart defect and accounts for 20% to 30% of all heart lesions.

Nursing process step: Assessment

Client needs category: Physiological integrity

Client needs subcategory: Physiological adaptation

Cognitive level: Application

9. The nurse is preparing to give an I.M. injection into the left leg of a 2-year-old. Identify the area where the nurse would give the injection.

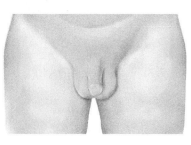

ANSWER:

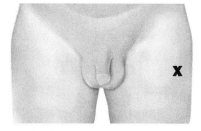

X

Rationale: The vastus lateralis muscle, located in the thigh, is the muscle into which the nurse should administer an I.M. injection into the leg of a toddler. To give an injection into the vastus lateralis muscle, the nurse should divide the distance between the greater trochanter and the knee joints into quadrants. The injection should be given in the center of the upper quadrant.

Nursing process step: Implementation

Client needs category: Physiological integrity

Client needs subcategory: Pharmacological and parenteral therapies

Cognitive level: Application

The preschooler

1. A nurse is caring for a 5-year-old who is in the terminal stages of cancer. Which statements are true?

Select all that apply:

☐ **A.** The parents may be at different stages in dealing with the child's death.

☐ **B.** The child is thinking about the future and knows he may not be able to participate.

☐ **C.** The dying child may become clingy and act like a toddler.

☐ **D.** Whispering in the child's room will help the child to cope.

☐ **E.** The death of a child may have long-term disruptive effects on the family.

☐ **F.** The child doesn't fully understand the concept of death.

ANSWER: A, C, E, F

Rationale: When dealing with a dying child, parents may be at different stages of grief at different times. The child may regress in his behaviors. The stress of a child's death commonly results in divorce and behavioral problems in siblings. Preschoolers see death as temporary—a type of sleep or separation. They recognize the word "dead" but don't fully understand its meaning. Thinking about the future is typical of an adolescent facing death, not a preschooler. Whispering in front of the child only increases his fear of death.

Nursing process step: Analysis

Client needs category: Psychosocial integrity

Client needs subcategory: Coping and adaptation

Cognitive level: Analysis

2. A 44-lb preschooler is being treated for inflammation. The physician orders 0.2 mg/kg/day of dexamethasone (Decadron) by mouth to be administered every 6 hours. The elixir comes in a strength of 0.5 mg/5 ml. How many milliliters of dexamethasone should the nurse give this client per dose?

_____

ANSWER: 10

Rationale: To perform this dosage calculation, the nurse should first convert the child's weight from pounds to kilograms:

$$44 \text{ lb} \div 2.2 \text{ lb/kg} = 20 \text{ kg}$$

Then she should calculate the total daily dose for the child:

$$20 \text{ kg} \times 0.2 \text{ mg/kg/day} = 4 \text{ mg}$$

Next, the nurse should calculate the amount to be given at each dose:

$$4 \text{ mg} \div 4 \text{ doses} = 1 \text{ mg/dose}$$

The available elixir contains 0.5 mg of drug per 5 ml. Therefore, to give 1 mg of the drug, the nurse should administer 10 ml to the child for each dose.

Nursing process step: Implementation

Client needs category: Physiological integrity

Client needs subcategory: Pharmacological and parenteral therapies

Cognitive level: Analysis

---

3. The nurse is performing a Denver Developmental Screening Test II on a 4½-year-old child. What behaviors should the nurse expect the child to demonstrate?

Select all that apply:

☐ **A.** He balances on each foot for at least 6 seconds.

☐ **B.** He copies a square using straight lines and square corners.

☐ **C.** He prepares his own cereal without help.

☐ **D.** He copies a circle that's closed or very nearly closed.

☐ **E.** He speaks clearly.

☐ **F.** He draws a person with at least three body parts.

ANSWER: C, D, E, F

Rationale: By age 4½, a child should be able to prepare a bowl of cereal without help, copy a circle, speak clearly, and draw a person using at least three body parts. The majority of children don't achieve balancing on each foot for 6 seconds until about age 5½. Less than 25% of all children are able to correctly copy a square by age 4.

Nursing process step: Analysis

Client needs category: Health promotion and maintenance

Client needs subcategory: Growth and development through the life span

Cognitive level: Analysis

4. A 4-year-old child has recently been diagnosed with acute lymphocytic leukemia (ALL). What information about ALL should the nurse provide when educating the client's parents?

Select all that apply:

☐ **A.** Leukemia is a rare form of childhood cancer.

☐ **B.** ALL affects all blood-forming organs and systems throughout the body.

☐ **C.** Because of the increased risk of bleeding, the child shouldn't brush his teeth.

☐ **D.** Adverse effects of treatment include sleepiness, alopecia, and stomatitis.

☐ **E.** There's a 95% chance of obtaining remission with treatment.

☐ **F.** The child shouldn't be disciplined during this difficult time.

ANSWER: B, D, E

Rationale: In ALL, abnormal white blood cells proliferate, but they don't mature past the blast phase. These blast cells crowd out the healthy white blood cells, red blood cells, and platelets in the bone marrow, leading to bone marrow depression. The blast cells also infiltrate the liver, spleen, kidneys, and lymph tissue. Common adverse effects of chemotherapy and radiation include nausea, vomiting, diarrhea, sleepiness, alopecia, anemia, stomatitis, mucositis, pain, reddened skin, and increased susceptibility to infection. There's a 95% chance of obtaining remission with treatment. Leukemia is the most common form of childhood cancer. The child still needs appropriate discipline and limits. A lack of consistent parenting may lead to negative behaviors and fear.

Nursing process step: Implementation

Client needs category: Physiological integrity

Client needs subcategory: Reduction of risk potential

Cognitive level: Application

---

5. A critically ill 4-year-old is in the pediatric intensive care unit. Telemetry monitoring reveals junctional tachycardia. Identify where this arrhythmia originates.

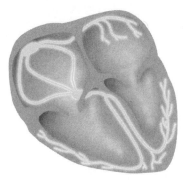

ANSWER:

Rationale: In junctional tachycardia, the atrioventricular node rapidly fires.

Nursing process step: Assessment

Client needs category: Physiological integrity

Client needs subcategory: Physiological adaptation

Cognitive level: Analysis

6. A 4-year-old is being treated for status asthmaticus. His arterial blood gas analysis reveals a pH of 7.28, P_{CO_2} of 55 mm Hg, and HCO_3^- of 26 mEq/L. What condition do these findings indicate?

_____

ANSWER: Respiratory acidosis

Rationale: A pH less than 7.35 and a Pa_{CO_2} greater than 45 mm Hg indicate respiratory acidosis. Status asthmaticus is a medical emergency that's characterized by respiratory distress. Persistent hypoventilation leads to the accumulation of carbon dioxide, resulting in respiratory acidosis.

Nursing process step: Analysis

Client needs category: Physiological integrity

Client needs subcategory: Physiological adaptation

Cognitive level: Analysis

---

7. A 4-year-old child is brought to the emergency department in cardiac arrest. The staff performs cardiopulmonary resuscitation (CPR). Identify the area where the child's pulse should be checked.

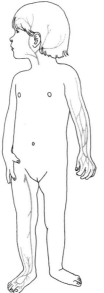

ANSWER:

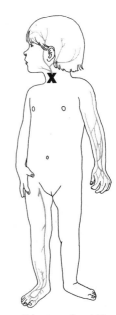

Rationale: The carotid artery should be used to check for a pulse when performing CPR on children and adults. The brachial pulse should be used when performing CPR on an infant.

Nursing process step: Assessment

Client needs category: Physiological integrity

Client needs subcategory: Physiological adaptation

Cognitive level: Application

---

8. A preschooler is scheduled to have a Wilm's tumor removed. Identify the area of the urinary system where a Wilm's tumor is located.

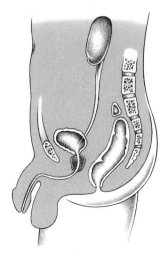

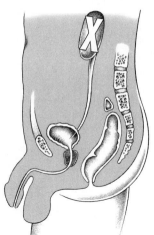

Rationale: A Wilm's tumor, also known as a *nephroblastoma,* is a tumor located on the kidney. It's most commonly found in children ages 2 to 4.

Nursing process step: Assessment

Client needs category: Physiological integrity

Client needs subcategory: Physiological adaptation

Cognitive level: Application

---

9. A 4½-year-old is ordered to receive 25 ml/hour of I.V. solution. The nurse is using a pediatric microdrip chamber to administer the medication. For how many drops per minute should the microdrip chamber be set?

ANSWER: 25

Rationale: When using a pediatric microdrip chamber, the number of milliliters per hour equals the number of drops per minute. If 25 ml/hour is ordered, the I.V. should infuse at 25 drops/minute.

Nursing process step: Implementation

Client needs category: Physiological integrity

Client needs subcategory: Pharmacological and parenteral therapies

Cognitive level: Application

1. A 7-year-old child is admitted to the hospital for a course of I.V. antibiotics. What should the nurse do before inserting the peripheral I.V. catheter?

Select all that apply:

☐ **A.** Explain the procedure to the child immediately before the procedure.

☐ **B.** Apply a topical anesthetic to the I.V. site before the procedure.

☐ **C.** Ask the child which hand he uses for drawing.

☐ **D.** Explain the procedure to the child using abstract terms.

☐ **E.** Don't let the child see the equipment to be used in the procedure.

☐ **F.** Tell the child that the procedure won't hurt.

ANSWER: B, C

Rationale: Topical anesthetics reduce the pain of a venipuncture. The cream should be applied about 1 hour before the procedure and requires a physician's order. Asking which hand the child draws with helps to identify the dominant hand. The I.V. should be inserted into the opposite extremity so that the child can continue to play and to do homework with a minimum amount of disruption. Younger school-age children don't have the capability for abstract thinking. The procedure should be explained using simple words and definitions of unfamiliar terms should be provided. The child should have the procedure explained to him well before it takes place so that he has time to ask questions. Although the topical anesthetic will relieve some pain, there's usually some pain or discomfort involved in venipuncture, so the child shouldn't be told otherwise.

Nursing process step: Implementation

Client needs category: Health promotion and maintenance

Client needs subcategory: Growth and development through the life span

Cognitive level: Application

---

2. The nurse is teaching bicycle safety to a child and his parents. What protective device should the nurse tell the parents is most important in preventing or lessening the severity of brain injury related to bicycle crashes?

_____

ANSWER: Helmet

Rationale: A well-fitting helmet is the most important safety feature to stress to children and parents. According to the American Academy of Pediatrics, wearing a helmet correctly can prevent or lessen the severity of brain injuries resulting from bicycle crashes.

Nursing process step: Implementation

Client needs category: Physiological integrity

Client needs subcategory: Reduction of risk potential

Cognitive level: Application

3. A child with sickle cell anemia is being discharged after treatment for a crisis. Which instructions for avoiding future crises should the nurse provide to the client and his family?

Select all that apply:

☐ **A.** Avoid foods high in folic acid.

☐ **B.** Drink plenty of fluids.

☐ **C.** Use cold packs to relieve joint pain.

☐ **D.** Report a sore throat to an adult immediately.

☐ **E.** Restrict activity to quiet board games.

☐ **F.** Wash hands before meals and after playing.

ANSWER: B, D, F

Rationale: Fluids should be encouraged to prevent stasis in the blood stream, which can lead to sickling. Sore throats, and any other cold symptoms, should be promptly reported because they may indicate the presence of an infection, which can precipitate a crisis (red blood cells sickle and obstruct blood flow to tissues). Children with sickle cell anemia should learn appropriate measures to prevent infection, such as proper hand washing techniques and good nutrition practices. Folic acid intake should be encouraged to help support new cell growth; new cells replace fragile, sickled cells. Warm packs should be applied to provide comfort and relieve pain; cold packs cause vasoconstriction. The child should maintain an active, normal life. When the child experiences a pain crisis, he limits his own activity according to his pain level.

Nursing process step: Planning

Client needs category: Physiological integrity

Client needs subcategory: Reduction of risk potential

Cognitive level: Application

---

4. The nurse is preparing to administer I.V. methylprednisolone sodium succinate (Solu-Medrol) to a child who weighs 42 lb. The order is for 0.03 mg/kg I.V. daily. How many milligrams should the nurse prepare?

ANSWER: 0.6

Rationale: To perform this dosage calculation, the nurse should first convert the child's weight to kilograms:

$$44 \text{ lb} \div 2.2 \text{ kg/lb} = 20 \text{ kg}$$

Then she should use this formula to determine the dose:

$$20 \text{ kg} \times 0.03 \text{ mg/kg} = X \text{ mg}$$

$$X = 0.6 \text{ mg}$$

Nursing process step: Implementation

Client needs category: Physiological integrity

Client needs subcategory: Pharmacological and parenteral therapies

Cognitive level: Application

5. An 8-year-old child has just returned from the operating room after having a tonsillectomy. The nurse is preparing to do a postoperative assessment. The nurse should be alert for which signs and symptoms of bleeding?

Select all that apply:

☐ **A.** Frequent clearing of the throat

☐ **B.** Breathing through the mouth

☐ **C.** Frequent swallowing

☐ **D.** Sleeping at long intervals

☐ **E.** Pulse rate of 98 beats/minute

☐ **F.** Blood-red vomitus

ANSWER: A, C, F

Rationale: A classic sign of bleeding after tonsillectomy is frequent swallowing; this occurs because blood drips down the back of the throat, tickling it. Other signs include frequent clearing of the throat and vomiting of bright red blood. Vomiting of dark blood may be seen if the child swallowed blood during surgery but doesn't indicate postoperative bleeding. Breathing through the mouth is common because of dried secretions in the nares. Sleeping at long intervals is normal after receiving sedation and anesthesia. A pulse rate of 98 beats/minute is in the normal range for this age-group.

Nursing process step: Assessment

Client needs category: Physiological integrity

Client needs subcategory: Reduction of risk potential

Cognitive level: Application

---

6. A 6-year-old child is being discharged from the emergency department after being diagnosed with varicella (chickenpox). What over-the-counter medication should the nurse instruct the parents to avoid administering to the child?

_____

ANSWER: Aspirin

Rationale: Using aspirin during a viral infection has been linked to Reye's syndrome, a serious illness that can lead to brain damage and death in children. If the child requires medication for fever or discomfort, the nurse should recommend acetaminophen (Tylenol) or ibuprofen (Motrin).

Nursing process step: Planning

Client needs category: Physiological integrity

Client needs subcategory: Pharmacological and parenteral therapies

Cognitive level: Analysis

7. A mother brings her child to the pediatrician's office for evaluation of chronic stomach pain. The mother states that the pain seems to go away when she tells the child that he can stay home from school. The physician diagnoses school phobia. Which other behaviors or symptoms may present in the child with school phobia?

Select all that apply:

☐ **A.** Nausea

☐ **B.** Headaches

☐ **C.** Weight loss

☐ **D.** Dizziness

☐ **E.** Fever

Rationale: Children with school phobia commonly complain of vague symptoms, such as stomachaches, nausea, headaches, and dizziness, to avoid going to school. These symptoms typically don't occur on weekends. A careful history must be taken to identify a pattern of school avoidance. Signs such as weight loss and fever are more likely to have a physiological cause and are uncommon in the child with school phobia.

Nursing process step: Analysis

Client needs category: Psychosocial integrity

Client needs subcategory: Psychosocial adaptation

Cognitive level: Analysis

---

8. A 10-year-old child visits the pediatrician's office for his annual physical examination. When the nurse asks how he's doing, he becomes quiet and states that his grandmother died last week. Which statements by the client show that he understands the concept of death?

Select all that apply:

☐ **A.** "Death is irreversible and final."

☐ **B.** "All people must die."

☐ **C.** "My grandmother's death has been hard to understand."

☐ **D.** "My grandmother died because she was sick and nothing could make her better."

☐ **E.** "My grandmother is dead, but she'll come back."

☐ **F.** "My grandmother died because someone in the family did something bad."

Rationale: By age 10, most children know that death is irreversible and final. However, a child may still have difficulty understanding the specific death of a loved one. School-age children should be able to identify cause and effect relationships, such as when a terminal illness causes someone to die. Adolescents, not school-age children, understand that death is a universal process. Preschoolers see death as temporary and may think of death as a punishment.

Nursing process step: Planning

Client needs category: Health promotion and maintenance

Client needs subcategory: Growth and development through the life span

Cognitive level: Analysis

9. A child with sickle cell anemia is being treated for a crisis. The physician orders morphine sulfate (Duramorph) 2 mg I.V. The concentration of the vial is 10 mg/1 ml of solution. How many milliliters of solution should the nurse administer?

_____

Answer: 0.2

Rationale: The nurse should calculate the volume to be given using this equation:

$$2 \text{ mg}/X \text{ ml} = 10 \text{ mg}/1 \text{ ml}$$

$$10 X = 2$$

$$X = 0.2 \text{ ml}$$

Nursing process step: Implementation

Client needs category: Physiological integrity

Client needs subcategory: Pharmacological and parenteral therapies

Cognitive level: Application

The adolescent

1. The nurse is caring for an adolescent girl who was admitted to the hospital's medical unit after attempting suicide by ingesting acetaminophen (Tylenol). The nurse should incorporate which interventions into the care plan for this client?

Select all that apply:

☐ **A.** Limit care until the client initiates a conversation.

☐ **B.** Ask the client's parents if they keep firearms in their home.

☐ **C.** Ask the client if she's currently having suicidal thoughts.

☐ **D.** Assist the client with bathing and grooming as needed.

☐ **E.** Inspect the client's mouth after giving oral medications.

☐ **F.** Assure the client that anything she says will be held in strict confidence.

Answer: B, C, D, E

Rationale: Safety is the primary consideration when caring for suicidal clients. Because firearms are the most common method used in suicides, the client's parents should be encouraged to remove firearms from the home, if applicable. Safety also includes assessing for current suicidal ideation. In many cases, suicidal people are depressed and don't have the energy to care for themselves, so the client may need assistance with bathing and grooming. Because depressed and suicidal clients may hide pills in their cheeks, the nurse should inspect the client's mouth after giving oral medications. Rather than limit care, the nurse should try to establish a trusting relationship through nursing interventions and therapeutic communication. The client can't be assured confidentiality when self-destructive behavior is an issue.

Nursing process step: Planning

Client needs category: Psychosocial integrity

Client needs subcategory: Psychosocial adaptation

Cognitive level: Application

2. The nurse is teaching an adolescent with inflammatory bowel disease about treatment with corticosteroids. Which adverse effects are concerns for this client?

Select all that apply:

☐ **A.** Acne

☐ **B.** Hirsutism

☐ **C.** Mood swings

☐ **D.** Osteoporosis

☐ **E.** Growth spurts

☐ **F.** Adrenal suppression

ANSWER: A, B, C, D, F

Rationale: Adverse effects of corticosteroids include acne, hirsutism, mood swings, osteoporosis, and adrenal suppression. Steroid use in children and adolescents may cause delayed growth, not growth spurts.

Nursing process step: Implementation

Client needs category: Physiological integrity

Client needs subcategory: Pharmacological and parenteral therapies

Cognitive level: Application

---

3. The nurse is caring for a 17-year-old female client with cystic fibrosis who has been admitted to the hospital to receive I.V. antibiotic and respiratory treatment for exacerbation of a lung infection. The client has a number of questions about her future and the consequences of the disease. Which statements about the course of cystic fibrosis are true?

Select all that apply:

☐ **A.** Breast development is frequently delayed.

☐ **B.** The client is at risk for developing diabetes.

☐ **C.** Pregnancy and child-bearing aren't affected.

☐ **D.** Normal sexual relationships can be expected.

☐ **E.** Only males carry the gene for the disease.

☐ **F.** By age 20, the client should be able to decrease the frequency of respiratory treatment.

ANSWER: A, B, D

Rationale: Cystic fibrosis delays growth and the onset of puberty. Children with cystic fibrosis tend to be smaller than average size and develop secondary sex characteristics later in life. In addition, clients with cystic fibrosis are at risk for developing diabetes mellitus because the pancreatic duct becomes obstructed as pancreatic tissues are destroyed. Clients with cystic fibrosis can expect to have normal sexual relationships, but fertility becomes difficult because thick secretions obstruct the cervix and block sperm entry. Males and females carry the gene for cystic fibrosis. Pulmonary disease commonly progresses as the client ages, requiring additional respiratory treatment—not less.

Nursing process step: Analysis

Client needs category: Physiological integrity

Client needs subcategory: Physiological adaptation

Cognitive level: Analysis

4. The nurse is preparing to administer the first dose of tobramycin (Nebcin) to an adolescent with cystic fibrosis. The order is for 3 mg/kg I.V. daily in three divided doses. The client weighs 95 lb. What many milligrams should the nurse administer per dose?

_____

ANSWER: 43.2

_____

Rationale: To perform this dosage calculation, the nurse should first convert the client's weight to kilograms using this formula:

$$1 \text{ kg}/2.2 \text{ lb} = X \text{ kg}/95 \text{ lb}$$

$$2.2X = 95$$

$$X = 43.2 \text{ kg}$$

Then, she should calculate the client's daily dose using this formula:

$$43.2 \text{ kg} \times 3 \text{ mg/kg} = 129.6 \text{ mg}$$

Finally, the nurse should calculate the divided dose:

$$129.6 \text{ mg} \div 3 \text{ doses} = 43.2 \text{ mg/dose}$$

Nursing process step: Implementation

Client needs category: Physiological integrity

Client needs subcategory: Pharmacological and parenteral therapies

Cognitive level: Application

Part 5

Psychiatric and mental health nursing

1. A client becomes angry and belligerent toward the nurse after speaking on the phone with his mother. The nurse recognizes this as what coping mechanism?

ANSWER: Displacement

Rationale: Displacement is a coping mechanism in which a person transfers his feelings for one person toward another person who is less threatening.

Nursing process step: Assessment

Client needs category: Psychosocial integrity

Client needs subcategory: Psychosocial adaptation

Cognitive level: Comprehension

2. A client is presented with the treatment option of electroconvulsive therapy (ECT). After discussing the treatment with the staff, the client requests that a family member come in to help him decide whether or not to undergo this treatment. What principle does the nurse consider in supporting the client's right to self-determination and autonomy?

ANSWER: Informed consent

Rationale: A client may ask for a family member's assistance in the treatment decision-making process at any time. During these times, the nurse must recognize that the client isn't ready to give informed consent.

Nursing process step: Evaluation

Client needs category: Psychosocial integrity

Client needs subcategory: Psychosocial adaptation

Cognitive level: Application

3. A female client is admitted to the emergency department (ED) after being sexually assaulted. The nurse notes that the client is sitting calmly and quietly in the examination room and recognizes this behavior as a protective defense mechanism. What defense mechanism is the client exhibiting?

_____

ANSWER: Denial

Rationale: Denial is a protective and adaptive reaction to increased anxiety. It involves consciously disowning intolerable thoughts and impulses. This response is often seen in victims of sexual abuse.

Nursing process step: Assessment

Client needs category: Psychosocial integrity

Client needs subcategory: Psychosocial adaptation

Cognitive level: Comprehension

---

4. On the second day of hospitalization, the client is discussing with the nurse concerns about unhealthy family relationships. During the nurse-client interaction, the client changes the subject to a job situation. The nurse responds, "Let's go back to what we were just talking about." What therapeutic communication technique did the nurse use?

_____

ANSWER: Focusing

Rationale: The therapeutic communication technique used by the nurse to redirect a client back to the original topic of discussion is called focusing. Focusing fosters the client's self-control and helps avoid vague generalizations, so the client can accept responsibility for facing problems.

Nursing process step: Implementation

Client needs category: Psychosocial integrity

Client needs subcategory: Psychosocial adaptation

Cognitive level: Application

5. The nurse is explaining the Bill of Rights for psychiatric patients to a client who has voluntarily sought admission to an inpatient psychiatric facility. Which of the following rights should the nurse include in the discussion?

Select all that apply:

☐ **A.** Right to select health care team members

☐ **B.** Right to refuse treatment

☐ **C.** Right to a written treatment plan

☐ **D.** Right to obtain disability

☐ **E.** Right to confidentiality

☐ **F.** Right to personal mail

ANSWER: B, C, E, F

Rationale: An inpatient client usually receives a copy of the Bill of Rights for psychiatric patients, which includes options B, C, E, and F. However, a client in an inpatient setting cannot select health team members. A client may apply for disability as a result of a chronic, incapacitating illness; however, disability is not a patient right, and members of a psychiatric institution do not decide who should receive it.

Nursing process step: Implementation

Client needs category: Psychosocial integrity

Client needs subcategory: Coping and adaptation

Cognitive level: Application

---

6. In the ED, a client reveals to the nurse a lethal plan for committing suicide and agrees to a voluntary admission to the psychiatric unit. Which information will the nurse discuss with the client to answer the question, "How long do I have to stay here?"

Select all that apply:

☐ **A.** "You may leave the hospital at any time unless you are suicidal."

☐ **B.** "Let's talk more after the health team has assessed you."

☐ **C.** "Once you've signed the papers, you have no say."

☐ **D.** "Because you could hurt yourself, you must be safe before being discharged."

☐ **E.** "You need a lawyer to help you make that decision."

☐ **F.** "There must be a court hearing before you leave the hospital."

ANSWER: A, B, D

Rationale: A person who is admitted to a psychiatric hospital on a voluntary basis may sign out of the hospital unless the health care team determines that the person is harmful to himself or others. The health care team evaluates the client's condition before discharge. If there is reason to believe that the client is harmful to himself or others, a hearing can be held to determine if the admission status should be changed from voluntary to involuntary. Option C is incorrect because it denies the client's rights; option E is incorrect because the client doesn't need a lawyer to leave the hospital; and option F is incorrect because a hearing isn't mandated before discharge. A hearing is held only if the client remains unsafe and requires further treatment.

Nursing process step: Implementation

Client needs category: Psychosocial integrity

Client needs subcategory: Coping and adaptation

Cognitive level: Application

7. The nurse has developed a relationship with a client who has an addiction problem. Which information would indicate that the therapeutic interaction is in the working stage?

Select all that apply:

☐ **A.** The client addresses how the addiction has contributed to family distress.

☐ **B.** The client reluctantly shares the family history of addiction.

☐ **C.** The client verbalizes difficulty identifying personal strengths.

☐ **D.** The client discusses the financial problems related to the addiction.

☐ **E.** The client expresses uncertainty about meeting with the nurse.

☐ **F.** The client acknowledges the addiction's effects on the children.

ANSWER: A, C, F

Rationale: Options A, C, and F are examples of the nurse-client working phase of an interaction. In the working phase, the client explores, evaluates, and determines solutions to identified problems. Options B, C, and E address what happens during the introductory phase of the nurse-client interaction.

Nursing process step: Evaluation

Client needs category: Psychosocial integrity

Client needs subcategory: Psychosocial adaptation

Cognitive level: Analysis

Anxiety disorders

1. A client on the behavioral health unit tells the nurse that she experiences palpitations, trembling, and nausea while traveling outside her home alone. These symptoms have severely limited her ability to function and have caused her to avoid leaving home whenever possible. The nurse recognizes that this client has symptoms of what disorder?

ANSWER: Agoraphobia

Rationale: Agoraphobia is a phobia or fear and avoidance of open spaces accompanied by the concern that escape to safety would be difficult or embarrassing. It's commonly accompanied by physical symptoms, such as palpitations, trembling, nausea, and shortness of breath. It's also commonly accompanied or preceded by panic attacks.

Nursing process step: Assessment

Client needs category: Psychosocial integrity

Client needs subcategory: Coping and adaptation

Cognitive level: Analysis

2. A client on the behavioral health unit confides in a nurse that she was raped 5 months before. During the nurse's assessment of her sleep patterns, the client complains of having difficulty falling and staying asleep. She attributes her irritability to sleep deprivation. Further questioning reveals that the client can't recall details of the rape, and feels detached when she has sex with her husband. The nurse recognizes that this client is experiencing symptoms of what disorder?

_____

ANSWER: Posttraumatic stress disorder

Rationale: Posttraumatic stress disorder (PTSD) is characterized by a pattern of symptoms resulting from exposure to a traumatic event. These symptoms last more than a month, distinguishing this client's disorder from acute stress disorder, which resolves within a month. Common symptoms of PTSD include intense fear, helplessness, or horror related to the trauma; recurrent and disturbing recollections or dreams of the trauma; avoidance of situations related to the trauma, symptoms of arousal such as difficulty falling or staying asleep; irritability; and an exaggerated startle response.

Nursing process step: Assessment

Client needs category: Psychosocial integrity

Client needs subcategory: Coping and adaptation

Cognitive level: Analysis

3. A client on the behavioral health unit spends several hours a day organizing and reorganizing his closet. He repeatedly checks to see if his clothing is arranged in the proper order. What term is commonly used to describe this behavior?

_____

ANSWER: Compulsion

Rationale: Compulsion is present when a client exhibits recurrent, persistent repetitive actions and behaviors, which he feels driven to perform. This behavior interferes with the client's activities of daily living and is disruptive to the client's lifestyle. These compulsions relieve the intense anxiety that occurs when the behavior isn't performed.

Nursing process step: Assessment

Client needs category: Psychosocial integrity

Client needs subcategory: Coping and adaptation

Cognitive level: Analysis

4. A client with the nursing diagnosis of *Fear, related to being embarrassed in the presence of others* exhibits symptoms of social phobia. What should the goals be for this client?

Select all that apply:

☐ **A.** Manage her fear in group situations.

☐ **B.** Develop a plan to avoid situations that may cause stress.

☐ **C.** Verbalize feelings that occur in stressful situations.

☐ **D.** Develop a plan for responding to stressful situations.

☐ **E.** Deny feelings that may contribute to irrational fears.

☐ **F.** Use suppression to deal with underlying fears.

Answer: A, C, D

Rationale: Improving stress management skills, verbalizing feelings and anticipating and planning for stressful situations are adaptive responses to stress. Avoidance, denial, and suppression are maladaptive defense mechanisms.

Nursing process step: Planning

Client needs category: Psychosocial integrity

Client needs subcategory: Coping and adaptation

Cognitive level: Application

---

5. The nurse recognizes improvement in a client with the nursing diagnosis of *Ineffective role performance related to the need to perform rituals*. Which of the following behaviors indicates improvement?

Select all that apply:

☐ **A.** The client refrains from performing rituals during stress.

☐ **B.** The client verbalizes that he uses "thought stopping" when obsessive thoughts occur.

☐ **C.** The client verbalizes the relationship between stress and ritualistic behaviors.

☐ **D.** The client avoids stressful situations.

☐ **E.** The client rationalizes ritualistic behavior.

☐ **F.** The client performs ritualistic behaviors in private.

Answer: A, B, C

Rationale: Refraining from rituals demonstrates that the client manages stress appropriately. Using "thought stopping" demonstrates the client's ability to employ appropriate interventions for obsessive thoughts. Verbalizing the relationship between stress and behaviors indicates that the client understands the disease process. Avoiding, rationalizing, and hiding behaviors demonstrate maladaptive methods for managing stress and anxiety.

Nursing process step: Evaluation

Client needs category: Psychosocial integrity

Client needs subcategory: Coping and adaptation

Cognitive level: Analysis

6. A recent diagnosis of cancer has caused a client severe anxiety. The nursing care plan should include which of the following interventions?

Select all that apply:

☐ **A.** Maintain a calm, non-threatening environment.

☐ **B.** Teach relevant aspects of chemotherapy.

☐ **C.** Encourage the client to verbalize her concerns regarding the diagnosis.

☐ **D.** Encourage the client to use deep-breathing exercises and other relaxation techniques during periods of increased stress.

☐ **E.** Provide distractions for the client during periods of stress.

☐ **F.** Teach the stages of grieving.

ANSWER: A, C, D

Rationale: During acute stress, interventions that help the client regain control will help the client master this new threat. Providing a calm, accepting attitude and encouraging verbalization of concerns will help the client face the unknown. Relaxation techniques have a physiologic and psychological effect in calming the client, which in turn allows further exploration of thoughts and feelings, as well as problem solving. Learning is limited during extreme stress so teaching wouldn't be effective at this stage. Providing distractions would be ineffective at this point in the grief process.

Nursing process step: Implementation

Client needs category: Psychosocial integrity

Client needs subcategory: Psychosocial adaptation

Cognitive level: Application

Mood, adjustment, and dementia disorders

1. At the request of his family, a client comes to a community mental health clinic for a psychiatric evaluation. During the initial interview, the client tells the nurse about painting the city streets to beautify them, lecturing about germ control to people riding the subway, and banning all people from smoking in order to clean up the environment. The client is irritable and easily distracted by the slightest sound. Which of the three stages of mania is the client exhibiting?

_____

ANSWER: Acute mania

Rationale: The client is demonstrating an expansive mood, high-energy level, racing thoughts, and disjointed thinking. Any type of stimulation will distract the client from the current conversation. This behavior is indicative of the acute manic phase of mania. The other two phases are hypomania and delirious mania.

Nursing process step: Assessment

Client needs category: Psychosocial integrity

Client needs subcategory: Coping and adaptation

Cognitive level: Analysis

2. During the nurse's assessment of a client who is depressed, the client reports that she's experiencing difficulty falling sleeping, a loss of appetite, and a decreased interest in sex. The nurse recognizes that the client is describing a lack of what type of activity?

_____

ANSWER: Vegetative

Rationale: Vegetative activities are those that promote health, and include eating, sleeping, elimination, and sex. Changes in these activities are commonly associated with depression.

Nursing process step: Analysis

Client needs category: Psychosocial integrity

Client needs subcategory: Coping and adaptation

Cognitive level: Analysis

---

3. In the community room, the nurse observes a client who suffers from depression. She sees the client pace swiftly around the room, swing both arms, and rub both hands together. What term would the nurse use to describe these behaviors to members of the health care team?

_____

ANSWER: Psychomotor agitation

Rationale: Psychomotor agitation is defined by constant motion, such as pacing, wringing hands, biting nails, and other types of energetic body movements.

Nursing process step: Assessment

Client needs category: Psychosocial integrity

Client needs subcategory: Coping and adaptation

Cognitive level: Analysis

4. During an interaction with the nurse, a client with bipolar disease states that she doesn't have anything to contribute to the art therapy group. Upon exploration of the client's concerns, the nurse recognized the client's pattern of withdrawal and non-participation in situations requiring communication with others. Which nursing diagnosis would be appropriate for this client?

_____

ANSWER: Impaired social interaction

Rationale: The data obtained by the nurse supports the nursing diagnosis of impaired social interaction. Some defining characteristics of this diagnosis include having limited communication with others, verbalizing negative feelings, and feeling insecure around other people.

Nursing process step: Analysis

Client needs category: Psychosocial integrity

Client needs subcategory: Psychosocial adaptation

Cognitive level: Analysis

---

5. After interviewing a client diagnosed with recurrent depression, the nurse determines the client's potential to commit suicide. Which factors would the nurse consider as contributors to the client's potential for suicide?

Select all that apply:

☐ **A.** Psychomotor retardation

☐ **B.** Impulsive behaviors

☐ **C.** Overwhelming feelings of guilt

☐ **D.** Chronic, debilitating illness

☐ **E.** Decreased physical activity

☐ **F.** Repression of anger

ANSWER: B, C, D, F

Rationale: Impulsive behavior, overwhelming guilt, chronic illness, and anger repression are factors that contribute to suicide potential. Psychomotor retardation and decreased activity are symptoms of depression, but don't typically lead to suicide because the client doesn't have the energy to harm himself.

Nursing process step: Analysis

Client needs category: Psychosocial integrity

Client needs subcategory: Psychosocial adaptation

Cognitive level: Analysis

6. The nurse is assessing a client who talks freely about feeling depressed. During the interaction, the nurse hears the client state, "Things will never change." What other indications of hopelessness would the nurse look for?

Select all that apply:

☐ **A.** Bouts of anger

☐ **B.** Periods of irritability

☐ **C.** Preoccupation with delusions

☐ **D.** Feelings of worthlessness

☐ **E.** Self-destructive behaviors

☐ **F.** Auditory hallucinations

ANSWER: A, B, D, E

Rationale: Clients who are depressed and feeling hopeless are often irritable and express inappropriate anger and suicidal thoughts. In addition, they may demonstrate self-destructive behaviors. Preoccupation with delusions and auditory hallucinations are generally seen in clients with schizophrenia or other psychotic disorders, rather than in those expressing hopelessness.

Nursing process step: Assessment

Client needs category: Psychosocial integrity

Client needs subcategory: Psychosocial adaptation

Cognitive level: Analysis

---

7. The nurse interviews the family of a client hospitalized with severe depression and suicidal ideation. What family assessment information is essential in formulating an effective plan of care?

Select all that apply:

☐ **A.** Physical pain

☐ **B.** Personal responsibilities

☐ **C.** Employment skills

☐ **D.** Communication patterns

☐ **E.** Role expectations

☐ **F.** Current family stressors

ANSWER: D, E, F

Rationale: When working with the family of a depressed client, it's helpful for the nurse to be aware of the family's communication style, the role expectations for its members, and current family stressors. This information can help to identify family difficulties and teaching points that could benefit the client and the family. Information concerning physical pain, personal responsibilities, and employment skills wouldn't be helpful because these areas aren't directly related to their experience of having a depressed family member.

Nursing process step: Planning

Client needs category: Psychosocial integrity

Client needs subcategory: Psychosocial adaptation

Cognitive level: Application

8. A client is prescribed sertraline (Zoloft), a selective serotonin reuptake inhibitor. Which information about this drug's adverse effects would the nurse include when creating a medication teaching plan?

Select all that apply:

☐ **A.** Agitation

☐ **B.** Agranulocytosis

☐ **C.** Sleep disturbance

☐ **D.** Intermittent tachycardia

☐ **E.** Dry mouth

☐ **F.** Seizures

Answer: A, C, E

Rationale: Common adverse effects of sertraline (Zoloft) are agitation, sleep disturbance, and dry mouth. Agranulocytosis, intermittent tachycardia, and seizures are adverse effects of clozapine (Clozaril).

Nursing process step: Planning

Client needs category: Physiological integrity

Client needs subcategory: Pharmacological and parenteral therapies

Cognitive level: Application

---

9. The nurse is assessing a client for dementia. What history would the nurse expect to find in a client with dementia?

Select all that apply:

☐ **A.** There is a slow progression of symptoms.

☐ **B.** The client admits to feelings of sadness.

☐ **C.** The client acts apathetic and pessimistic.

☐ **D.** The family can't determine when the symptoms first appeared.

☐ **E.** There are changes in the client's basic personality.

☐ **F.** The client has great difficulty paying attention to others.

Answer: A, D, E, F

Rationale: Common characteristics of dementia are a slow onset of symptoms, which makes it difficult to determine when symptoms first occurred. It progresses to noticeable changes in the individual's personality and impaired ability to pay attention to other people. Feelings of sadness, apathy, and pessimism are symptoms of depression.

Nursing process step: Analysis

Client needs category: Health promotion and maintenance

Client needs subcategory: Prevention and early detection of disease

Cognitive level: Analysis

10. A client has been diagnosed with an adjustment disorder with mixed anxiety and depression. What are the primary nursing diagnoses associated with an adjustment disorder?

Select all that apply:

☐ **A.** Activity intolerance

☐ **B.** Impaired social interaction

☐ **C.** Self-esteem disturbance

☐ **D.** Personal identity disturbance

☐ **E.** Acute confusion

☐ **F.** Impaired memory

ANSWER: B, C

Rationale: A client with an adjustment disorder is likely to have impaired social interaction and self-esteem disturbance. Activity intolerance, personal identity disturbance, acute confusion, and impaired memory aren't related to the diagnosis of adjustment disorder.

Nursing process step: Analysis

Client needs category: Psychosocial integrity

Client needs subcategory: Psychosocial adaptation

Cognitive level: Analysis

Psychotic disorders

1. A physician prescribes lithium for a client diagnosed with bipolar disorder. The nurse needs to provide appropriate education for the client on this drug. Which of the following topics should the nurse cover?

Select all that apply:

☐ **A.** The potential for addiction

☐ **B.** Signs and symptoms of drug toxicity

☐ **C.** The potential for tardive dyskinesia

☐ **D.** A low-tyramine diet

☐ **E.** The need to consistently monitor blood levels

☐ **F.** Changes in his mood that may take 7 to 21 days

ANSWER: B, E, F

Rationale: Client education should cover the signs and symptoms of drug toxicity as well as the need to report them to the physician. The client should be instructed to monitor his lithium levels on a regular basis to avoid toxicity. The nurse should explain that 7 to 21 days may pass before the client notes a change in his mood. Lithium does not have addictive properties. Tyramine is a potential concern to clients taking monoamine-oxidase inhibitors.

Nursing process step: Implementation

Client needs category: Physiological integrity

Client needs subcategory: Pharmacological and parenteral therapies

Cognitive level: Application

2. The nurse is monitoring a client who appears to be hallucinating. She notes paranoid content in the client's speech and he appears agitated. The client is gesturing at a figure on the television. Which of the following nursing interventions are appropriate?

Select all that apply:

☐ **A.** In a firm voice, instruct the client to stop the behavior.

☐ **B.** Reinforce that the client is not in any danger.

☐ **C.** Acknowledge the presence of the hallucinations.

☐ **D.** Instruct other team members to ignore the client's behavior.

☐ **E.** Immediately implement physical restraint procedures.

☐ **F.** Use a calm voice and simple commands.

ANSWER: B, C, F

Rationale: Using a calm voice, the nurse should reassure the client that he is safe. She shouldn't challenge the client; rather, she should acknowledge his hallucinatory experience. It is not appropriate to request that the client stop the behavior. Implementing restraints is not warranted at this time. Although the client is agitated, no evidence exists that the client is at risk for harming himself or others.

Nursing process step: Implementation

Client needs category: Psychosocial integrity

Client needs subcategory: Psychosocial adaptation

Cognitive level: Application

---

3. A client with schizophrenia is taking the atypical antipsychotic medication clozapine (Clozaril). Which of the following signs and symptoms indicate the presence of adverse effects associated with this medication?

Select all that apply:

☐ **A.** Sore throat

☐ **B.** Pill-rolling movements

☐ **C.** Polyuria

☐ **D.** Fever

☐ **E.** Polydipsia

☐ **F.** Orthostatic hypotension

ANSWER: A, D

Rationale: Sore throat, fever, and sudden onset of other flulike symptoms are signs of agranulocytosis. The condition is caused by a lack of a sufficient number of granulocytes (a type of white blood cell), which causes the individual to be susceptible to infection. The client's white blood cell count should be monitored at least weekly throughout the course of treatment. Pill-rolling movements can occur in those experiencing extrapyramidal adverse effects associated with antipsychotic medication that has been prescribed for much longer than a medication such as clozapine. Polydipsia (excessive thirst) and polyuria (increased urine) are common adverse effects of lithium. Orthostatic hypotension is an adverse effect of tricyclic antidepressants.

Nursing process step: Assessment

Client needs category: Physiological integrity

Client needs subcategory: Pharmacological therapies

Cognitive level: Application

4. A delusional client approaches the nurse, stating, "I am the Easter bunny," and insisting that the nurse refer to him as such. The belief appears to be fixed and unchanging. Which of the following nursing interventions should the nurse implement when working with this client?

Select all that apply:

☐ **A.** Consistently use the client's name in interaction.

☐ **B.** Smile at the humor of the situation.

☐ **C.** Agree that the client is the Easter Bunny.

☐ **D.** Logically point out why the client could not be the Easter Bunny.

☐ **E.** Provide an as-needed medication.

☐ **F.** Provide the client with structured activities.

ANSWER: A, F

Rationale: Continued reality-based orientation is necessary, so it is appropriate to use the client's name in any interaction. Structured activities can help the client refocus and resolve his delusion. The nurse shouldn't contribute to the delusion by going along with the situation. Logical arguments and an as-needed medication aren't likely to change the client's beliefs.

Nursing process step: Implementation

Client needs category: Psychosocial integrity

Client needs subcategory: Coping and adaptation

Cognitive level: Analysis

---

5. A physician starts a client on the antipsychotic medication haloperidol (Haldol). The nurse is aware that this medication has extrapyramidal adverse effects. Which of the following measures should the nurse take during Haldol administration?

Select all that apply:

☐ **A.** Review subcutaneous injection technique.

☐ **B.** Closely monitor vital signs, especially temperature.

☐ **C.** Provide the client with the opportunity to pace.

☐ **D.** Monitor blood glucose levels.

☐ **E.** Provide the client with hard candy.

☐ **F.** Monitor for signs and symptoms of urticaria.

ANSWER: B, C, E

Rationale: Neuroleptic malignant syndrome is a life-threatening extrapyramidal adverse effect of antipsychotic medications such as Haldol. It's associated with a rapid increase in temperature. The most common extrapyramidal adverse effect, akathisia, is a form of psychomotor restlessness that can often be relieved by pacing. Haldol and the anticholinergic medications that are provided to alleviate its extrapyramidal effects can result in dry mouth. Providing the client with hard candy to suck on can help alleviate this problem. Haldol isn't given subcutaneously and doesn't affect blood glucose levels. Urticaria is not usually associated with Haldol administration.

Nursing process step: Planning

Client needs category: Physiological integrity

Client needs subcategory: Pharmacological and parenteral therapies

Cognitive level: Analysis

6. The nurse observes that a client diagnosed with schizophrenia is staring into space and doesn't acknowledge the presence of others. At times, the client moves rapidly but then stops and remains in one posture for long periods. What form of schizophrenia is the nurse observing?

_____

ANSWER: Catatonic

Rationale: A client with catatonic schizophrenia shows a lack of responsiveness to the environment. The client may move rapidly or slowly, often alternating between patterns of movement. In many cases, he then poses and appears rigid. The other forms of schizophrenia—paranoid, disorganized, undifferentiated, and residual—are associated with different patterns of behavior and responses. However, disruption of motor behavior in conjunction with a lack of responsiveness to the immediate environment occurs only in the catatonic form of schizophrenia.

Nursing process step: Assessment

Client needs category: Psychosocial integrity

Client needs subcategory: Psychosocial adaptation

Cognitive level: Knowledge

7. A client with schizophrenia displays a lack of interest in activities, reduced affect, and poor ability to perform activities of daily living (ADLs). What term would be used to describe this clustering of symptoms?

_____

ANSWER: Negative

Rationale: Schizophrenic clients often display positive and negative symptoms. Negative symptoms are characterized by the absence of typically displayed emotional responses. Clients with these symptoms tend to respond poorly to medication. Positive symptoms, such as auditory or visual hallucinations, are characterized by enhancement of a sensory modality.

Nursing process step: Assessment

Client needs category: Psychosocial integrity

Client needs subcategory: Psychosocial adaptation

Cognitive level: Knowledge

8. One of the causes of schizophrenia involves an overstimulation of what neurotransmitter?

_____

ANSWER: Dopamine

Rationale: Studies on the role of neurotransmitters in schizophrenia have identified that the disease results (at least in part) from an overactive dopamine system in the brain. Excessive dopamine activity may be responsible for such symptoms as hallucinations, agitation, delusional thinking, and grandiosity—forms of hyperactivity that have been linked to excessive dopamine activity.

Nursing process step: Assessment

Client needs category: Physiological integrity

Client needs subcategory: Physiological adaptation

Cognitive level: Knowledge

Substance abuse, eating disorders, and impulse control disorders

1. An adolescent client is being admitted to the psychiatric unit for treatment of an eating disorder. Her admission interview reveals a history of recurrent episodes of binge eating and self-induced vomiting. The nurse recognizes these as symptoms of what disease?

_____

ANSWER: Bulimia nervosa

Rationale: The essential features of bulimia nervosa include eating binges followed by feelings of guilt, humiliation, and self-deprecation. These feelings cause the client to engage in self-induced vomiting, use laxatives or diuretics, follow a strict diet, or fast to overcome the effects of the binges.

Nursing process step: Assessment

Client needs category: Psychosocial integrity

Client needs subcategory: Psychosocial adaptation

Cognitive level: Analysis

2. The nurse is assessing a client with a history of multiple substance abuse. The client reports that he's been experiencing nausea, vomiting, and diarrhea. The nurse observes flushing, piloerection (hair erection), increased lacrimation (secretion of tears), and rhinorrhea. These signs and symptoms most likely indicate withdrawal from what category of drugs?

_____

ANSWER: Opioid

Rationale: Typical symptoms of opioid addiction and withdrawal include flushing, piloerection, nausea, vomiting, abdominal cramps, increased lacrimation, and rhinorrhea. The nurse must be alert for symptoms of opioid withdrawal due to an increase in abuse of opioids, such as heroine and hydrocodone.

Nursing process step: Assessment

Client needs category: Psychosocial integrity

Client needs subcategory: Psychosocial adaptation

Cognitive level: Analysis

---

3. The nurse is assisting in the discharge planning for a client with alcoholism. To what outpatient support group should she refer the client?

_____

ANSWER: Alcoholics Anonymous

Rationale: Alcoholics Anonymous is an outpatient support group for recovering alcoholics. It allows clients to share their problems and gain support from members of the group to avoid further alcohol abuse.

Nursing process step: Planning

Client needs category: Safe, effective care environment

Client needs subcategory: Coordinated care

Cognitive level: Analysis

4. The nurse is caring for an anorexic client with a nursing diagnosis of *Imbalanced nutrition: Less than body requirements* related to dysfunctional eating patterns. Which of the following interventions would be supportive for this client?

Select all that apply:

☐ **A.** Provide small, frequent meals.

☐ **B.** Monitor weight gain.

☐ **C.** Allow the client to skip meals until the antidepressant levels are therapeutic.

☐ **D.** Encourage the client to keep a journal.

☐ **E.** Monitor the client during meals and for 1 hour after meals.

☐ **F.** Encourage the client to eat three substantial meals per day.

ANSWER: A, B, D, E

Rationale: Due to self-starvation, clients with anorexia rarely can tolerate large meals three times per day. Small, frequent meals may be tolerated better by the client with anorexia and they provide a way to gradually increase daily caloric intake. The nurse should monitor the client's weight carefully because a client with anorexia may try to hide weight loss. The client may be emotionally restrained and afraid to express her feelings; keeping a journal can serve as an outlet for these feelings, which can assist recovery. A client with anorexia is already underweight and shouldn't be permitted to skip meals.

Nursing process step: Implementation

Client needs category: Psychosocial integrity

Client needs subcategory: Psychosocial adaptation

Cognitive level: Analysis

---

5. When assessing a client diagnosed with impulse control disorder, the nurse observes violent, aggressive, and assaultive behavior. Which of the following assessment data is the nurse also likely to find?

Select all that apply:

☐ **A.** The client functions well in other areas of his life.

☐ **B.** The degree of aggressiveness is out of proportion to the stressor.

☐ **C.** The violent behavior is most often justified by a stressor.

☐ **D.** The client has history of parental alcoholism and chaotic abusive family life.

☐ **E.** The client has no remorse about the inability to control his behavior.

ANSWER: A, B, D

Rationale: A client with an impulse control disorder who display violent, aggressive, and assaultive behavior generally functions well in the other areas of his life. The degree of aggressiveness is out of proportion to the stressor and he frequently has a history of parental alcoholism and a chaotic family life. The client often verbalizes sincere remorse and guilt for the aggressive behavior.

Nursing process step: Assessment

Client needs category: Psychosocial integrity

Client needs subcategory: Psychosocial adaptation

Cognitive level: Application

6. The nurse is planning care for a client who has a history of making verbal threats and acting violently toward, including throwing objects at, family members. The client is currently displaying intense anger towards the staff. What nursing diagnosis is most appropriate?

_____

ANSWER: Risk for other-directed violence

Rationale: A history of violence, threats, violent antisocial behavior, and threatening body language all suggest the nursing diagnosis of _Risk for other-directed violence._

Nursing process step: Analysis

Client needs category: Psychosocial integrity

Client needs subcategory: Psychosocial adaptation

Cognitive level: Application

---

7. A client is receiving chlordiazepoxide (Librium) to control the symptoms of alcohol withdrawal. The chlordiazepoxide has been ordered as needed. Which of the following symptoms may indicate the need for an additional dose of this medication?

Select all that apply:

☐ **A.** Tachycardia

☐ **B.** Mood swings

☐ **C.** Elevated blood pressure and temperature

☐ **D.** Piloerection

☐ **E.** Tremors

☐ **F.** Increasing anxiety

ANSWER: A, C, E, F

Rationale: Benzodiazepines are usually administered based on elevations in heart rate, blood pressure, and temperature as well as on the presence of tremors and increasing anxiety. Mood swings are expected during the withdrawal period and are not an indication for further medication administration. Piloerection is not a symptom of alcohol withdrawal.

Nursing process step: Evaluation

Client needs category: Physiological integrity

Client needs subcategory: Pharmacological and parenteral therapies

Cognitive level: Analysis